Therapeutics

Nadia Bukhari
Masters of Pharmacy Programme Manager and
Preregistration Co-ordinator, School of Pharmacy,
University of London, UK

David Kearney
Senior Pharmacist in Neurology,
University Hospitals of Leicester NHS Trust,
Leicester, UK

Pharmaceutical Press

Published by Pharmaceutical Press

66-68 East Smithfield, London E1W 1AW, UK

© Pharmaceutical Press 2009

(**PP**) is a trade mark of Pharmaceutical Press

Pharmaceutical Press is the publishing division of the Royal
Pharmaceutical Society of Great Britain

First published 2009
Reprinted 2010, 2012, 2013, 2014

Typeset by Thomson Digital, Noida, India
Printed in Great Britain by TJ International, Padstow, Cornwall

ISBN 978 0 85369 775 6

A catalogue record for this book is available from the British Library.

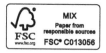

FASTtrack

Therapeutics

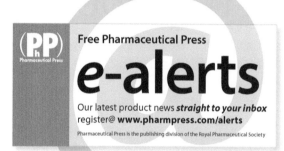

Dedication

I would like to dedicate this book to my beautiful daughter Myra Bukhari, my pride and joy

Nadia Bukhari

I would like to dedicate this book to all those who have helped me throughout my journey of life

David Kearney

Contents

Introduction to the *FASTtrack* series

FASTtrack is a new series of revision guides created for undergraduate pharmacy students. The books are intended to be used in conjunction with textbooks and reference books as an aid to revision to help guide students through their examinations. They provide essential information required in each particular subject area. The books will also be useful for pre-registration trainees preparing for the Royal Pharmaceutical Society of Great Britain's (RPSGB's) registration examination, and to practising pharmacists as a quick reference text.

The content of each title focuses on what pharmacy students really need to know in order to pass exams. Features include*:
- concise bulleted information
- key points
- tips for the student
- multiple choice questions (MCQs) and worked examples
- case studies
- simple diagrams.

The titles in the *FASTtrack* series reflect the full spectrum of modules for the undergraduate pharmacy degree.

Future titles include:
Pharmaceutical Compounding and Dispensing
Physical Pharmacy (based on Florence & Attwood's *Physicochemical Principles of Pharmacy*)
Managing Symptoms in the Pharmacy
Pharmaceutics – Dosage Form and Design
Pharmaceutics – Drug Delivery and Targeting
Complementary and Alternative Medicine
Pharmacology

*Note: not all features are in every title in the series.

About the authors

NADIA BUKHARI worked as a pharmacy manager at Westbury Chemist, Streatham for a year after qualifying, after which she moved on to work for Barts and the London NHS Trust as a clinical pharmacist in surgery. It was at this time that she developed an interest in teaching, as part of her role involved responsibility as a teacher practitioner for the School of Pharmacy, University of London.

Two and a half years later, she commenced working for the School of Pharmacy, University of London, as the Preregistration Co-ordinator for the school and the academic facilitator, which involved teaching therapeutics to MPharm students and assisting the Director of Undergraduate Studies.

Nadia currently has the role of the Masters of Pharmacy Programme Manager, which involves management of the undergraduate degree.

Nadia's interest in therapeutics emerged from teaching at undergraduate level and completing her postgraduate diploma in pharmacy practice, hence the stimulus to write this book.

DAVID KEARNEY undertook his pre-registration training at the University Hospitals of Leicester after graduating from the University of Manchester. He continued his training as a rotational junior pharmacist at Barts and the London NHS Trust. He remained there for several years, specialising in a number of areas, including respiratory medicine, HIV and GUM, and infection management. In 2007, he became Clinical Lecturer at the School of Pharmacy, University of London, teaching clinical pharmacy for a number of undergraduate and postgraduate courses.

In the summer of 2008, he relocated back to Leicester and took up a post as a Senior Pharmacist in Neurology.

Acknowledgements

The authors wish to acknowledge the support received from students and colleagues at the School of Pharmacy, University of London.

We especially thank our parents and families for their encouragement and unconditional faith in us.

We would also like to express thanks to the editors at the Pharmaceutical Press, who have been very supportive, especially the senior commissioning editor Christina De Bono for her guidance.

Finally, we wish to thank our spouses – Murtaza and Laura – for putting up with the late nights and providing continuous support, making this book possible.

Introduction

Therapeutics is a branch of medicine that is related to the application of drugs and other remedies for preventing, curing or healing disease.

Many aspects should be considered when determining the appropriateness of therapy for patients (Figure 0.1).

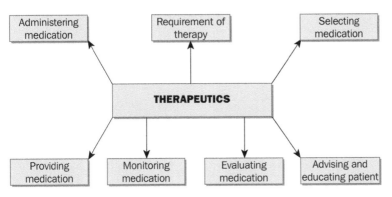

Figure 0.1

Each chapter will explore a different medical condition and involve the aspects outlined above. By focusing on the key points of each disease state, this book aims to provide the reader with a concise overview of therapeutics.

How the book is laid out

The book is organised into 33 chapters, arranged into 10 sections based on body systems (e.g. gastrointestinal) or types of condition (e.g. infectious diseases). Each chapter is structured in the same way to provide a systematic approach and facilitate learning.

- Key points
- Aetiology: the causes of the disease/condition
- Epidemiology: the incidence and prevalence of the disease/condition
- Signs and symptoms: usual signs and symptoms that the patient will have on presentation
- Investigations: tests and examinations used to confirm a diagnosis
- Management: non-drug treatment and drug treatment available for the management of the disease/condition
- Monitoring parameters: features requiring monitoring for the efficacy and toxicity of the proposed treatments

- Counselling: key points to inform the patients about their therapy
- Multiple choice questions: questions that can be used to assess the reader's understanding of the disease/condition.

In addition, useful hints and tips will be interspersed through the chapters.

chapter 1
Basic clinical biochemistry

Table 1.1 Biochemical and haematological reference ranges

Tests (serum/plasma/whole blood)	Reference range	Units	Sample
Alanine aminotransferase (ALT)	40	U/L	Serum
Albumin	35–50	g/L	Serum
Alkaline phosphatase (ALP)	39–117	U/L	Serum
Aspartate aminotransferase (AST)	12–39	U/L	Serum
Bicarbonate	22–29	mmol/L	Serum
Bilirubin (total)	17	μmol/L	Serum
Bilirubin (direct)	4	μmol/L	Serum
C reactive protein	10	mg/L	Serum
Calcium	2.15–2.65	mmol/L	Serum
Chloride	98–106	mmol/L	Serum
Cholesterol: recommended	5.2	mmol/L	Serum
Cholesterol population range	3.5–6.7	mmol/L	Serum
Cholesterol (HDL), male	0.8–1.8	mmol/L	Serum
Cholesterol (HDL), female	1.0–2.3	mmol/L	Serum
Cholesterol (LDL): recommended	4.0	mmol/L	Fasting serum
Creatinine, male	79–118	μmol/L	Serum
Creatinine, female	58–93	μmol/L	Serum
Creatinine clearance, male	95–140	mL/min	Serum/24 h urine
Creatinine clearance, female	85–125	mL/min	Serum/24 h urine
Ferritin, male	20–260	μg/L	Serum
Ferritin, female	6–110	μg/L	Serum
Gamma glutamyltransferase (GGT), males	58	U/L	Serum
Gamma glutamyltransferase (GGT), females	31	U/L	Serum
Glucose (fasting)	3.9–6.1	mmol/L	Fluoride, oxalate
Glycated haemoglobin (HbA1c)	3.7–5.1	%	EDTA
Iron, male	12–31	μmol/L	Serum
Iron, female	9–30	μmol/L	Serum
Magnesium	0.70–1.00	mmol/L	Serum
Parathormone (PTH)	1.1–6.8	pmol/L	Serum
Phosphate	0.8–1.5	mmol/L	Serum
Potassium	3.5–5.1	mmol/L	Serum
Sodium	136–146	mmol/L	Serum
Triglycerides	2.1	mmol/L	Fasting serum
Urea	2.5–6.4	mmol/L	Serum
Urea (70 years)	3.7–10.0	mmol/L	Serum

Table 1.2 Blood tests

Parameter	Normal range
White blood count (WBC)	
Adults	$4.0-11.0 \times 10^9/L$
Male	$4.5-6.5 \times 10^{12}/L$
Female	$3.8-5.8 \times 10^{12}/L$
Haemoglobin	
Male	13.5–17.5 g/dL (135–175 g/L)
Female	11.5–16.5 g/dL (115–165 g/L)
Haematocrit	
Male	0.400–0.540
Female	0.370–0.470
Mean cell volume (MCV), adults	80–96 fL
Mean cell haemoglobin (MCH), adults	27.0–32.0 pg
Mean cell haemoglobin concentration (MCHC), adults and children	32.0–36.0 g/dL
Platelets, adults and children	$150-400 \times 10^9/L$
Erythrocyte sedimentation rate (ESR) Westergren method	
Male	1–10 mm in 1 h
Female	3–15 mm in 1 h

Table 1.3 Differential white cell count

White cells	Adults ($\times 10^9/L$)
Neutrophils	2.00–7.50
Lymphocytes	1.50–4.00
Monocytes	0.20–0.80
Eosinophils	0.04–0.40
Basophils	0.01–0.10

Table 1.4 Haemostasis tests

	Reference range
Prothrombin time (INR, PTR)	1.0–1.3 (ratio)
Activated partial thromboplastin time (KPTT)	23–31 s
Vitamin B_{12}	179–1132 ng/L
Red cell folate	149–640 μg/L
Serum folate	2.9–18.0 μg/L

INR, international normalised ratio; PTR, prothrombin time; KPTT, kaolin partial thromboplastin time.

Sodium

Sodium is responsible for maintaining osmolality of serum.

Hypernatraemia

Causes
- Water loss: inadequate water intake or excessive loss
- Sodium gain: increased sodium intake or decreased excretion

- Drugs, e.g. oral contraceptives, lactulose, corticosteroids, sodium bicarbonate and IV fluids.

Signs and symptoms
- Muscle weakness
- Raised jugular venous pressure
- Pulmonary oedema
- Signs of dehydration: thirst, confusion
- Decreased skin turgor.

Treatment
- Hypernatraemia from water loss: replace water
- Hypernatraemia from excess sodium gain: treatment with diuretics and water recommended
- Drug-induced hypernatraemia: discontinue therapy and seek alternative.

Hyponatraemia

Causes
- Water retention: syndrome of inappropriate secretion of antidiuretic hormone (SIADH) or renal impairment
- Sodium depletion: increased loss of sodium from the kidney, gut or skin
- Drugs, e.g. amphotericin, carbamazepine, lithium, non-steroidal anti-inflammatory drugs (NSAIDs), opiates.

Tip

It is extremely rare to have depleted sodium levels as a result of inadequate intake of sodium.

Signs and symptoms
- Sodium depletion: dizziness, dry mucous membranes, increased pulse, postural hypotension, decreased urine output, decreased consciousness and decreased skin turgor
- Water retention: signs and symptoms usually absent, although some may experience signs of oedema.

Treatment
- Sodium depletion: replace with sodium and water, preferably orally
- Water retention: oedema, if present, is treated with diuretics and restricted fluids; if oedema absent, restrict fluids
- Drug induced: discontinue therapy and seek alternative.

Potassium

Potassium is the predominant intracellular cation. Its main roles include regulating cardiac function and fluid balance.

Hyperkalaemia

Causes

- Renal failure: potassium accumulation from reduced excretion by damaged kidney
- Acidosis: redistribution of potassium into the extracellular fluid space
- Cell damage: potassium releasing as it is an intracellular ion.

Signs and symptoms

- Muscle weakness
- Cardiac arrest.

Treatment

- Infusion of insulin and glucose: shifts potassium ions into the cells
- Calcium gluconate infusion: counteracts effects of hyperkalaemia
- Dialysis: used only in severe hyperkalaemia
- Cation-exchange resins (calcium resonium): used in instances where the rise in potassium is slow and steady.

Hypokalaemia

Causes

- Drug induced: diuretics and corticosteroids
- Alkalosis: shifts potassium from the extracellular fluid to the intracellular fluid
- Gastrointestinal (GI): vomiting and diarrhoea may cause potassium loss
- Renal: increased aldosterone production.

Signs and symptoms

- Severe muscle weakness
- Cardiac arrythmias.

Treatment

Potassium salts: given orally or intravenously.

Phosphate

Phosphate is widespread in the body. Most is found in bone. Phosphate has a critical role in transferring, storing and utilising energy in the body.

Hyperphosphataemia

Causes
- Renal failure: decreased excretion by a damaged kidney
- Cell damage: releasing phosphate ions
- Hypoparathyroidsm: low parathormone decreases phosphate excretion, resulting in accumulation of the ion.

Tip

Calcium and phosphate have a mutual relationship; if one rises, the other falls. For example, if serum phosphate rises, serum calcium will fall.

Signs and symptoms
There are no relevant signs and symptoms.

Hypophosphataemia

Causes
- Alkalosis: shifting of phosphate ions into the cells
- Antacids: preventing the absorption of phosphate ions in the GI tract (e.g. aluminium hydroxide).

Signs and symptoms
Muscle weakness leading to respiratory impairment.

Treatment
Intravenous infusion of phosphate.

Magnesium

Over 300 enzyme systems are activated by magnesium; it is a very important intracellular cation.

Hypermagnesaemia
Hypermagnesaemia is uncommon but may be seen in renal impairment.

Hypomagnesaemia
Magnesium is present in most common foods. A deficiency may occur if dietary intake is low.

Signs and symptoms
- Tetany
- Tremor
- Convulsions
- Muscle weakness.

Treatment

Administration of oral or IV magnesium. Foods rich in magnesium include artichokes, bananas, wheat, nuts, spinach and pumpkin seeds.

Multiple choice questions

1. **Are the following statements regarding sodium true or false?**
a. Hyponatraemia may be caused by drugs.
b. Hypernatraemia symptoms include thirst.
c. Sodium is responsible for maintaining osmolality of serum.
d. If oedema is present in hyponatraemia, diuretics may be indicated.

2. **Are the following statements regarding ions in the body true or false?**
a. Hyperkalaemia may lead to cardiac arrest if untreated.
b. Hyperphosphataemia may be caused by damage to cells.
c. Magnesium has little value in the serum, its excess or loss has little effect.
d. Hypokalaemia can be caused by loop diuretics.

The cardiovascular system

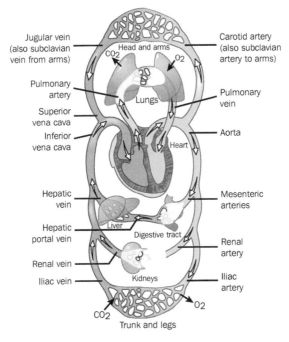

Figure 2.1 The cardiovascular system.

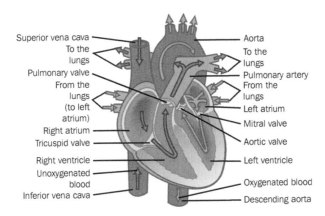

Figure 2.2 The heart.

Overview

- Hypertension (high blood pressure) is a condition where the blood pressure is consistently above 140/90 mmHg.
- Hypertension is usually asymptomatic.
- The aim of treatment is to reduce blood pressure and minimise cardiovascular risk.
- Lifestyle changes can reduce blood pressure and cardiovascular risk.
- Five main classes of drugs are used for treatment of hypertension; all work by reducing blood pressure: angiotensin-converting enzyme (ACE) inhibitors, calcium-channel blockers, thiazide diuretics, beta-blockers and alpha-blockers.

Tip

Drug therapy should be given to patients with persistent high blood pressure above 160/100 mmHg or persistent blood pressure above 140/90 mmHg and raised cardiovascular risk.

Aetiology

- Hypertension (high blood pressure) is a condition where the blood pressure is consistently above 140/90 mmHg.
- 90–95% of patients suffer from essential hypertension; with unknown cause.
- 5–10% of patients suffer with secondary hypertension, which is a consequence of a disease or drugs.

Essential hypertension

- Family history: blood pressure usually runs in families and children of hypertensive individuals are often affected.
- Obesity: overweight individuals have higher blood pressures than thinner individuals.
- Sodium intake: individuals with high salt consumption have higher blood pressures than those with lower sodium intake.
- Stress: acute pain and stress have been known to elevate blood pressure.

Secondary hypertension

- Pregnancy
- Alcohol
- Renal diseases
- Coarctation of the aorta
- Endocrine diseases, e.g. Conn's disease, Cushing's disease, acromegaly, hyperparathyroidism
- Drugs, e.g. combined oral contraceptives, NSAIDs, steroids, sympathomimetics.

Epidemiology

Risk factors associated with hypertension are:

- age: hypertension is more common in the elderly as blood pressure increases with age
- race: Black people of Afro-Caribbean origin are more likely to suffer with hypertension.

Signs and symptoms

- Hypertension is usually asymptomatic.
- Headaches have been reported by some patients.

Tip

In the UK, all patients under the age of 80 should have their blood pressure checked every 5 years.

Investigations

Most patients are diagnosed at routine check-ups or when a complication arises.

- Hypertension should be diagnosed using a validated device which has been maintained regularly.
- If the first reading exceeds 140/90 mmHg, then another reading should be taken at the end of the appointment.
- The blood pressure of both arms should be taken; the value from the arm with the higher reading is used as the baseline.
- Patients with confirmed diagnosis should be monitored monthly.

Tip

To confirm diagnosis of hypertension, the patient should return for two subsequent appointments and at least two measurements should be taken at each appointment.

The following tests should also be carried out to assess cardiovascular risk:
- urinalysis for protein
- plasma glucose
- electrolytes
- creatinine
- serum total and high-density lipoprotein (HDL)cholesterol
- 12-lead electrocardiography (ECG).

Management

- Aim of treatment is to reduce blood pressure and minimise cardiovascular risk.
- The target blood pressure to achieve is 140/90 mmHg or less.
- Treatment is based on the guidelines of the British Hypertension Society and the National Institute for Health and Clinical Excellence (NICE).
- Lifestyle adjustments by the patient should be tried before initiating drug treatment (Table 2.1).

Tip

Daily salt intake should be 6 g sodium chloride or 100 mmol sodium.

Table 2.1 Lifestyle changes

	Changes
Diet	Factors improving cardiovascular risk: eat healthy, well-balanced meals; five portions of fruit and vegetables a day; minimise caffeine drinks
Exercise	In patients who are overweight, weight loss reduces blood pressure
Alcohol	Reduced alcohol intake should be encouraged if drinking excessively
Smoking	Stopping smoking can reduce cardiovascular risk and cardiac events

Drug classes for hypertension

Five main classes of drug are used for treatment of hypertension; all work by reducing blood pressure

Tip

Therapy with a single drug is recommended initially; however, more drugs can be added to achieve target blood pressure.

- *Angiotensin-converting enzyme (ACE) inhibitors* block the conversion of angiotensin I to angiotension II (potent vasoconstrictor) resulting in vasodilatation.
- *Calcium-channel blockers* block slow calcium channels in the peripheral blood vessels and heart; the dihydropyridines (used in hypertension) work by decreasing peripheral resistance.
- *Thiazide diuretics* reduce circulating blood volume and decrease peripheral resistance.
- *Beta-blockers* reduce cardiac output.
- *Alpha-blockers* reduce total peripheral resistance and blood pressure.

Figure 2.3 shows the recommendations of the British Hypertension Society for combining blood pressure-lowering drugs.

Monitoring parameters

Tip

ACE inhibitors can cause a rapid fall in blood pressure in patients taking concurrent diuretic therapy, due to volume depletion; caution is advised.

ACE inhibitors

Examples are captopril, enalapril and ramipril.
- Monitor blood pressure as ACE inhibitors can cause profound hypotension.
- Renal function should be monitored as renal impairment may occur.
- ACE inhibitors inhibit the breakdown of bradykinin, causing a persistent dry cough in some patients.
- Other side-effects to watch out for are angioedema, rash, hyperkalaemia, GI effects and altered liver function tests.

Angiotensin II receptor antagonists are useful alternatives to ACE inhibitors in patients who suffer with the dry cough. These drugs do not inhibit the breakdown of bradykinin, which causes the dry cough and commonly disrupts ACE inhibitor therapy.

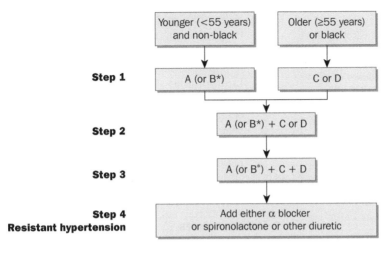

Younger (<55 years) and non-black	Older (≥55 years) or black

Step 1   A (or B*) | C or D

Step 2   A (or B*) + C or D

Step 3   A (or B*) + C + D

Step 4
Resistant hypertension   Add either α blocker or spironolactone or other diuretic

A: ACE inhibitor or angiotensin
   receptor blocker
B: β blocker

C: Calcium channel blocker
D: Diuretic (thiazide and
   thiazide-like)

* Combination therapy involving B and D may induce more new onset diabetes compared with other combination therapies

Figure 2.3 British Hypertension Society guidelines for hypertension management 2004 (BHS-IV): recommendations for combining blood pressure lowering drugs (AB/CD rule). (From Williams *et al.* (2004). *Br Med J* 328: 634–640; http://www.bhsoc.org/pdfs/Summary%20Guidelines%202004.pdf.)

Calcium-channel blockers

Examples are amlodipine, diltiazem, verapamil and nifedipine.

- All calcium-channel blockers cause hypotension, facial flushing and oedema.
- Each calcium-channel blocker has its own set of side-effects, which need to be monitored (see *British National Formulary* (BNF) Section 2.6.2).
- Verapamil should *not* be used with beta-blockers as it can cause heart block.

There are two types of calcium-channel blockers, dihydropyridines and negative inotropes (verapamil and diltiazem), with differing effects on the heart:

- dihydropyridines relax vascular smooth muscle and have less influence on the heart
- verapamil and diltiazem reduce cardiac output and slow heart rate.

Thiazide diuretics

Example is bendroflumethiazide.

- Diuretics are well tolerated in most patients.

Tip

For the management of hypertension, a low-dose thiazide is given. Bendroflumethiazide is used at a dose of 2.5 mg as it produces a maximal blood pressure-lowering effect with minimal side-effects.

- Side-effects include postural hypotension, hypokalaemia (monitor potassium ions), hypomagnesaemia (monitor magnesium) hyponatraemia (monitor sodium).
- Lipid profiles should be monitored as altered plasma lipid concentrations may occur.
- Watch for signs of gout as thiazides may cause hyperuricaemia, predisposing the patient to gout.
- Blood glucose levels should be monitored, especially if the patient has diabetes as thiazides may cause hyperglycaemia.

Tips

Both lipid-soluble and water-soluble beta-blockers can cause vivid dreams. However, this is less of a problem with the water-soluble beta-blockers, such as atenolol.

Beta-blockers are to be used with caution in diabetic patients as they can mask the effects of hypoglycaemia.

Beta-blockers

Examples are propranolol and atenolol. The use of beta-blockers in hypertension is decreasing as they seem less effective in preventing stroke and cardiac events.

- Monitoring parameters include pulse, as beta-blockers may cause bradycardia, and blood pressure, as hypotension may occur.
- Side-effects to monitor include coldness of extremities, fatigue, vivid dreams, sexual dysfunction, bradycardia and bronchospasm.
- Beta-blockers (including the cardioselective ones) are contraindicated in asthmatics as they can cause bronchospasm.

Alpha-blockers

Examples are doxasozin and phentolamine.
- Profound postural hypotension may occur with first dose.
- Side-effects to monitor include dizziness, fatigue and GI disturbances.

Counselling

- Patients should be counselled on lifestyle changes.
- Medication should be taken every day as advised and not stopped unless advised by the doctor or pharmacist.
- Patients should be aware of the side-effects of the drugs they are taking and report any disturbing side-effects to their pharmacist or doctor.
- An annual review of blood pressure should be provided and patients can be counselled on monitoring their own blood pressure.

Multiple choice questions

1. **Hypertension is when the blood pressure is persistently over:**
a. 120/80 mmHg
b. 130/80 mmHg
c. 140/90 mmHg
d. 130/90 mmHg
e. 140/80 mmHg

2. **Are the following statements true or false?**
a. Beta-blockers should be used with caution in diabetic patients.
b. ACE inhibitors are the antihypertensive drug of choice in diabetic patients.
c. Thiazide diuretics are not recommended in the elderly.
d. Verapamil should not be given with beta-blockers.

Useful websites

http://www.nice.org.uk
http://www.bhsoc.org

chapter 3
Angina

Overview

- Angina is a chronic condition characterised by recurrent chest pain or discomfort brought about by exertion or stress.
- It is caused by inadequate perfusion of the myocardium as a result of atherosclerosis or vasospasm.
- Treatment aims to reduce symptoms and reduce the incidence of more serious coronary artery disease.
- Beta-blockers are the first-line treatment in the majority of patients.
- Many patients will require interventional procedures to provide adequate relief of symptoms.

Aetiology

- Stable angina is a clinical syndrome that is a chronic form of coronary heart disease (CHD).
- Angina presents when the coronary blood supply cannot meet the demand of the myocardium.
- The resulting mild ischaemia causes the symptoms of angina.
- The reason for the reduction in coronary blood supply is usually atherosclerosis, or, occasionally, coronary artery spasms.
- While at rest, there is usually an adequate blood flow to the myocardium; however, under stress, such as exercise, the blockage prevents an adequate blood flow and results in the characteristic symptoms.
- Angina caused by spasm of the coronary arteries is known as Prinzmetal angina. In this condition, symptoms may occur at rest as well as under exertion. It is usually treated with calcium-channel blockers or nitrates.

Epidemiology

- There are 92 000 new cases diagnosed annually in the UK.
- Angina is more common in males, with 54% of newly diagnosed cases.
- Prevalence increases with age; in those aged 55–64 years, there is a prevalence of 8% in men and 3% in women, and in those aged 65–74 years, there is a prevalence of 14% in men and 8% in women.
- It is estimated that there are over 1.1 million people in the UK with angina.

Tips

- The incidence is greater in those of South-East Asian origin than the general UK population, while it is lower in those of Afro-Caribbean origin.
- 10% of patients will suffer a myocardial infarction during the first year after diagnosis.
- The *risk factors* are similar to those for myocardial infarction and include:
  - smoking
  - diabetes
  - high plasma cholesterol
  - hypertension
  - stress
  - alcohol
  - increasing age
  - male sex.

Signs and symptoms

The presentation of angina may vary between patients; however, most will report the main symptom of chest discomfort precipitated by exertion.

Other symptoms include:
- tight, dull or heavy feeling of discomfort
- discomfort that is retrosternal or left sided in nature, radiating to the left arm, neck, jaw or back
- breathlessness
- relief of symptoms on rest.

Other triggers may include cold weather, large meals or emotional stress.

Investigations

Tip

- Diagnosis is made by assessing clinical symptoms and history, and confirming with objective assessments.
- An initial assessment should include assessment of blood pressure, cholesterol levels, blood glucose, thyroid function tests and haemoglobin.
- Patients should also receive a baseline electroencephalogram (ECG).
- A diagnosis of angina can be confirmed using a number of methods:
  - exercise tolerance tests
  - coronary angiography

- myocardial perfusion scintigraphy
- stress echocardiography.

■ Coronary angiography is regarded as the definitive test as it demonstrates the presence of occlusions, their position and their severity. This technique uses a catheter inserted into the patient's arterial circulation to inject radio-opaque dye into the coronary arteries. This is then visualised using sophisticated X-ray imaging.

Management

■ The management of angina focuses on:
- reducing the symptoms of the condition
- preventing progression of the condition
- reducing the risk of severe cardiovascular events.

■ Drug therapy used for prevention of anginal symptoms aims to reduce myocardial oxygen demand or improve coronary blood supply, and includes beta-blockers, calcium-channel blockers, nitrates, nicorandil and ivabridine.

■ *Beta-blockers* are considered first-line treatment for angina:
- they reduce heart rate and force of contraction, allowing greater time for perfusion and decreased demand for oxygen
- cardioselective beta-blockers, such as atenolol and metoprolol, are preferred
- all may cause bronchoconstriction in those with reversible airways disease, such as asthma
- other agents may be used as add-on therapy in those with inadequate response to beta-blockers or as an alternative to beta-blockers in those who have contraindications or are intolerant.

■ *Calcium-channel blockers* cause vasodilatation, increasing blood supply to the myocardium. Rate-limiting calcium-channel blockers also decrease oxygen demand:
- rate-limiting calcium-channel blockers, such as verapamil, should be avoided in most patients receiving beta-blockers owing to the risk of asystole, but are used when the patient is not receiving beta-blockers
- in those receiving beta-blockers and remaining symptomatic, the addition of a dihydropyridine-type calcium-channel blocker (e.g. nifedipine or amlodipine) is usually the next step.

■ *Nitrates* cause vasodilatation through the release of nitric oxide:

Tip

Aspirin is used to prevent cardiovascular events in those with heart disease, such as angina. It works through inhibition of cyclo-oxygenase. It is thought that other cyclo-oxygenase inhibitors, such as NSAIDs, may reduce its efficacy through competitive binding of active sites. As such, aspirin should be taken prior to any NSAIDs the patient is taking.

- significant first pass metabolism affects oral therapy, so for rapid effect nitrates are given via alternative routes such as sublingually
- short-acting nitrates, such as sublingual glyceryl trinitrate spray or tablets, are used for the rapid relief of symptoms of angina or the prevention of symptoms prior to exercise
- long-acting nitrates, such as isosorbide mononitrate, are taken orally and provide long-term prevention of symptoms.

■ *Nicorandil* is a potassium channel activator that causes coronary artery vasodilatation. Less is known about the long-term benefits of nicorandil than for the other agents.

■ *Ivabridine* is a new class of antianginal drug that affects the hyperpolarisation-activated current (I_f) channel current. Its place in therapy is not fully determined but it may be a useful alternative in those unable to receive beta-blockers.

■ All patients should be considered for antiplatelet and statin therapy to help to prevent progression of the condition.

■ *Antiplatelet* drugs include aspirin and clopidogrel. Both are effective in preventing cardiovascular events in those with conditions such as angina. The choice of agent is usually determined by cost or patient factors, such as previous intolerance to aspirin.

■ *Statins* lower cholesterol but are also thought to have antithrombotic and anti-inflammatory properties. They have benefits even in those with 'normal' cholesterol.

■ The addition of an ACE inhibitor, while having no effect on anginal symptoms, may decrease the risk of cardiovascular events.

■ In those who fail to respond to drug therapy, or where there is occlusion of numerous coronary arteries or the left main stem artery, coronary artery bypass graft (CABG) surgery or percutaneous coronary intervention (PCI) should be considered:

- CABG surgery utilises patent blood vessels from elsewhere in the patient's body to provide an alternative blood supply to the patient's myocardium
- in PCI, a balloon attached to a catheter in used to open the patient's coronary vessels (angioplasty), which may also be held open with a metal stent.

Tip

Patients should be counselled regarding the importance of a nitrate-free period. This may be achieved by utilising a dosing schedule where the two daily doses of long-acting nitrate are taken on waking and in the early afternoon.

Monitoring parameters

■ Patients should be regularly reviewed by their primary care team.

■ The incidence, frequency and severity of their symptoms should be assessed to determine the level of control.

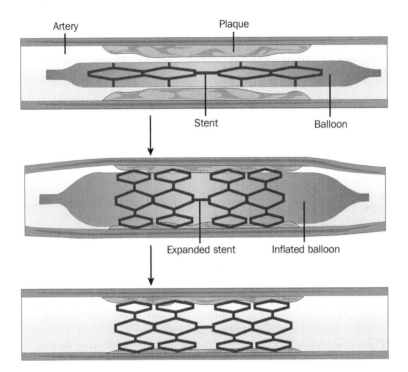

Figure 3.1 Placement and expansion of a stent in balloon angioplasty.

- In those with inadequate control despite optimisation of current therapy, an additional agent should be added.
- Those remaining symptomatic despite optimisation of two concurrent agents should be referred to secondary care for further assessment and management, which may include invasive non-pharmacological methods.
- Patients should also be assessed for the presence of drug-related adverse effects.
- Beta-blockers may cause peripheral vasoconstriction, leading to cold extremities, lethargy and fatigue, and dream disturbances.
- Nitrates may cause headaches, hypotension and dizziness. Tolerance may also develop with continual use. Hence, a nitrate-free period is utilised during the period of lowest risk, usually during the night.
- Calcium-channel blockers can cause constipation, flushing and ankle oedema.
- Nicorandil is generally well tolerated but may cause headache.

- Ivabridine may cause headache, dizziness and visual disturbances.
- Assessment and optimisation of other risk factors should also be undertaken.

Counselling

- Patients should be aware of their condition, its symptoms and its potential to cause more significant cardiovascular events.
- They should know how to recognise the signs of myocardial infarction.
- They should receive counselling to help them to address their other cardiovascular risk factors, such as smoking cessation and weight reduction.
- Education on the importance of appropriate exercise techniques should also be provided.
- Their drug regimen should be fully explained, including dosing, indication and potential adverse effects.
- Detailed counselling should be provided on the optimal use of their nitrate-relieving medication, with particular care paid to the method of administration (e.g. sublingual).
- Beta-blockers should not be stopped abruptly owing to the potential for rebound symptoms.
- Nicorandil can affect the ability to drive or operate machinery.

> ## Tip
>
> It is extremely important that patients are able to differentiate between their normal angina symptoms and those of potentially more serious events, such as myocardial infarction, as their outcome is likely to be better the faster they receive treatment for these. They should be told to dial 999 if their symptoms last longer than 5 min and are unresponsive to glyceryl trinitrate.

Multiple choice questions

1. Which of the following is *not* a recognised treatment for the prevention of angina symptoms?
a. Atenolol
b. Verapamil
c. Ivabridine
d. Ramipril
e. Nicorandil

2. Are the following statements true or false?
a. Beta-blockers are considered the first-line treatment of angina unless contraindicated.
b. Patients should be considered for statin treatment even if they have normal cholesterol levels.
c. Metoprolol and amlodipine should be avoided owing to the risk of asystole.

d. It is usual for the symptoms of angina to last for up to 15 min.
e. Angina is associated with a significantly increased risk of myocardial infarction.

Useful websites

www.sign.ac.uk
www.bhf.org.uk

chapter 4
Heart failure

Overview

- Heart failure is a common condition that results in insufficient cardiac output to meet the body's needs.
- Its incidence increases with age and it results in significant mortality and morbidity.
- The target of drug therapy is the overstimulation of the sympathetic nervous system and the renin–angiotensin–aldosterone system.
- Drug therapy consists of beta-blockers and ACE inhibitors in all stages of the disease and the use of other agents for the management of symptoms.

Aetiology

- Heart failure is the inability of the heart to attain the circulatory demands of the body.
- A healthy heart, at rest, undertakes 70 beats/min, each with a stroke volume of 70 mL; this results in a cardiac output of almost 5 L.
- When full, the left ventricle contains 130 mL of blood, meaning that the usual ejection fraction is over 50%.
- In heart failure, the ejection fraction is lower, with symptoms occurring more commonly with further decreases and becoming likely at an ejection fraction of 35%.
- Increased cardiac afterload results in hypertrophy of the cardiac muscles, leading to increased workload and decreased ejection fraction.
- Reduced blood flow to the heart (e.g. from ischaemic damage after myocardial infarction) causes impairment in the function of cardiac muscle.
- In response to circulatory failure, the body undertakes haemodynamic and neurohormonal changes.
- There is stimulation of the sympathetic nervous system and the renin–angiotensin–aldosterone system (RAAS), which results in increased vascular resistance and venous return.
- Increased sympathetic activity increases the heart rate but also leads to arrhythmias.
- Increased activity of RAAS causes an increase in circulatory volume, resulting in renal impairment. This leads to water and sodium retention and further activation of RAAS.

> **Tip**
>
> Right-sided heart failure is much less common than left sided and is caused by chronic lung disease, cor pulmonale. The management is not as understood and consists mainly of symptomatic relief with diuretics.

- Increased aldosterone activity also leads to myocardial fibrosis, causing stiffening of cardiac muscle.
- This cycle of increased activation and decreased cardiac output results in the symptoms and complications of heart failure.

Epidemiology

- Prevalent is 0.3–2/100 in the general population but rises to 10/100 in those aged over 65 years.
- The incidence doubles with each decade over 45 years of age.
- Incidence is increasing because of better mortality outcomes in myocardial infarction and an increasing population.
- The median survival from diagnosis is approximately 5 years, with wide variations dependent on the cause and severity of the heart failure.
- In the USA, Afro-Caribbean individuals have a greater incidence and mortality from heart failure than Whites.
- 70% of heart failure is thought to be caused by hypertension or ischaemic heart disease. Other causes may be alcohol abuse, anaemia, pregnancy, thyrotoxicosis and infection.
- Heart failure may result from drug therapy, for example anthracycline chemotherapy, excessive IV fluid replacement, corticosteroids and NSAIDs (causing fluid retention).

Signs and symptoms

There are many signs and symptoms of heart failure, some of which are used in the diagnosis and classification of severity of the condition. They result from decreased cardiac output and include:

- oedema
- dyspnoea
- orthopnoea
- hypoxia
- cough, often with sputum with may be frothy or blood stained
- fatigue
- cold extremities
- decreased exercise tolerance
- weight loss, although weight gain may occur with increased oedema
- tachycardia
- pallor
- confusion
- decreased urine output
- dizziness.

The New York Heart Association classification is used to assess the severity of heart failure:[1]

stage 1: asymptomatic undertaking normal activity

stage 2: slight limitation from dyspnoea on moderate or severe exertion, such as walking up hills or stairs

stage 3: marked limitations from dyspnoea on normal exertion

stage 4: dyspnoea at rest.

Investigations

Because there is a wide variety of causes and symptoms of heart failure and there is no definitive test, a range of investigations must be undertaken in those with suspected heart failure.

■ Blood tests:
– full blood to investigate anaemia
– creatinine, urea and electrolytes to assess renal function
– blood glucose to assess likelihood of diabetes
– arterial blood gases
– thyroid and liver function tests
– plasma brain natriuretic peptide, which may indicate heart failure.
■ Echocardiography can help to determine the cause and severity of heart disease: it may be used to determine left ventricular systolic function, diastolic function, severity of hypertrophy, valve function and pulmonary artery systolic pressure.
■ Chest radiography can assess enlargement of heart and whether any lung problems could be contributing to breathlessness.
■ Urinalysis assesses renal dysfunction and diabetes mellitus.
■ ECG assesses the presence of any other cardiac problems, such as arrhythmias.

> **Tip**
>
> No one test currently exists that can be used to determine the presence of heart failure. A detailed clinical history and thorough investigations must be undertaken to make a definitive diagnosis.

Management

The main goals of therapy are to:
■ relieve symptoms
■ improve exercise tolerance
■ reduce progression
■ reduce mortality.

This is done through using drug therapy to decrease cardiac workload, increase output and counteract the adaptive changes.

■ It is widely recommended that all patients with heart failure, regardless of severity receive an *ACE inhibitor* and a *beta-blocker*, unless contraindicated or not tolerated.

> **Tip**
>
> While the efficacy of ACE inhibitors is thought to be a class effect, the activity of beta-blockers varies significantly between agents so the latter are not interchangeable in heart failure.

- The maximum tolerated dose of each drug should be used.
- ACE inhibitors are initiated first, generally, but beta-blockers could be initiated before ACE inhibitors depending on patient factors.
- Beta-blockers should only be initiated in those with stable heart failure.
- Beta-blockers reduce the influence of the sympathetic nervous system in heart failure. Bisoprolol and carvedilol are widely used in the UK, with metoprolol succinate used in other countries. Nebivolol is indicated in the management of stable mild to moderate heart failure in those over 70 years of age.
- The effect of ACE inhibitors is thought to be a class effect so any may be used. They work by reducing pre- and afterload on the heart, resulting in increased cardiac output.
- *Angiotensin II receptor antagonists* may be used in those with intolerance to ACE inhibitors. Candesartan may also be prescribed by specialists in those remaining symptomatic on ACE inhibitors and beta-blockers.
- *Diuretics* are commonly used to manage fluid overload and oedema. Thiazides may be used in mild disease but are ineffective if renal impairment is also present.
- Loop diuretics, such as furosemide, are used to induce diuresis.
- If single diuretics do not produce sufficient effect they may be combined. Metolazone is occasionally used because it has significant diuretic activity; however, caution must be exercised as there is a likelihood of electrolyte disturbances.
- *Aldosterone antagonists*, eplerenone and spironolactone, are indicated in those with class 2 to class 4 heart failure.
- *Digoxin* can be used in those in sinus rhythm when other options have been ineffective.
- A combination of hydralazine and isosorbide dinitrate has been shown to be beneficial in Afro-Caribbean patients.

Tip

Cardiac rehabilitation courses may be helpful for patients with classes 2 and 3. These help patients to regain confidence to undertake exercise under the guidance of trained professionals and in the presence of other patients with heart failure.

Monitoring parameters

- The presence and severity of heart failure symptoms should be regularly assessed to determine the efficacy of current therapy and the need for further treatment.
- All patients should also be regularly assessed for the presence of complications of the condition and their medication.
- ACE inhibitors may cause hypotension, which may be minimised by careful titrating of the dose from a low starting dose.
- Through deactivation of the RAAS, ACE inhibitors result in a mild, and insignificant, renal impairment in most patients. However, in

those with pre-existing renal artery stenosis, they may cause a significant reduction in renal function. Therefore, monitoring of creatinine and urea is necessary within 2 weeks of therapy initiation and after each dose adjustment.

- The presence of minor but discomforting adverse effects such as cough and rash should also be observed.
- Beta-blockers cause hypotension, and may also cause bradycardia, so monitoring of blood pressure and heart rate is necessary.
- Beta-blockers may cause a worsening in symptoms on initiation but benefit becomes apparent after a number of weeks.
- The adverse effects of angiotensin receptor antagonists are similar to those of ACE inhibitors, except that the incidence of cough is significantly less.
- Diuretics can result in electrolyte disturbances, especially hypokalaemia, so monitoring of electrolytes is essential. Monitoring patient's weight, breathlessness and peripheral oedema signs may be useful in assessing the effectiveness of therapy.
- Aldosterone antagonists may cause hyperkalaemia, especially when used with ACE inhibitors, so monitoring of electrolytes is necessary.
- Digoxin therapy should be reviewed regularly for effectiveness and stopped if the patient derives no benefit. Signs of toxicity should be monitored and plasma levels may be monitored to ensure suitable doses are used.

Counselling

- Patients should be fully educated to their condition, including the prognosis, treatment goals and the potential complications.
- They should be educated to appropriate lifestyle interventions, such as exercise programmes, smoking cessation and reductions in alcohol intake, diet and sodium intake.
- They should be educated to the purpose, dosing and potential adverse effects of their medications. Specific issues for each medication should be addressed.
- ACE inhibitors may cause cough, hypotension, taste disturbances, rash and dizziness.

Tips

The pharmacist can be a useful source of advice for patients.

Many over-the-counter medications may cause problems for those with heart failure. This is usually because of their sodium or potassium content, sodium retention or sympathomimetic activity (e.g. indigestion remedies, NSAIDs and laxatives). Patients with heart failure should be encouraged to check with their pharmacist prior to purchasing any over-the-counter medication.

Although fewer than 10% of patients experience a persistent, harmless cough with ACE inhibitors, it is one of the main problems with their use. The cough is often first recognised by community pharmacists on questioning patients asking for remedies for persistent cough.

- Beta-blockers may cause impotence, tiredness and worsening of symptoms on initiation, which may worry patients that do not expect them.
- Diuretics will cause diuresis, and timings of doses should be adapted to lifestyle. In some patients, variable doses may be used according to symptoms and weight changes.
- Digoxin may cause problems in toxic doses. Signs of toxicity include nausea, anorexia, diarrhoea, visual disturbances and confusion.
- Gynaecomastia may occur with spironolactone and, although harmless, can be uncomfortable for patients.

Multiple choice questions

1. **Are the following statements true or false?**
a. All patients with heart failure should receive an ACE inhibitor unless contraindicated.
b. The benefits of beta-blockers in heart failure are apparent within a few days of initiation.
c. A normal ejection fraction is 45%.
d. Spironolactone may cause hyperkalaemia.
e. Digoxin may be used for symptomatic relief, even in those without arrhythmias.

Reference

1. New York Heart Association (1994). *Nomenclature and Criteria for Diagnosis of Diseases of the Heart and Great Vessels.* 9th edn. Boston, MA: Little, Brown and Co, 253–256.

Useful websites

www.nice.org.uk
www.sign.ac.uk
www.bhf.org.uk

chapter 5

Ischaemic heart disease

Overview

- Ischaemic heart disease is sometimes referred to as coronary heart disease.
- Acute coronary syndromes compose the most acute, and usually most fatal, episodes. These can be divided into unstable angina, non-ST elevation myocardial infarction and ST elevation myocardial infarction.
- Ischaemia is caused by full or partial occlusions of coronary arteries.
- Management is targeted at restoring patency of occluded vessels, providing symptomatic relief and preventing further occurrences.
- Modification of patient's risk factors may help to prevent further episodes.

Aetiology

- The underlying pathology of ischaemic heart disease (IHD) is the development of atherosclerosis within one or more coronary arteries leading to impaired blood flow or thromboembolic occlusion.
- Thromboembolic occlusions result in myocardial infarction, commonly known as 'heart attack'.
- Atherosclerosis, the formation of 'plaques', is thought to be the result of macrophages binding to the surface of coronary arteries and building up low-density lipoproteins.
- This initial stage is thought to be reversible; however, if it continues 'foam cells' are produced as cholesterol is incorporated from cell membranes.
- With increasing plaque size, cell death in the core results in a build up of lipid surrounded by a fibrin layer.
- The more lipid contained in a plaque, the more unstable it becomes.
- When a lipid-rich plaque erupts, the exposed lipids cause platelet activation and lead to the formation of thrombus.
- Total occlusion of coronary arteries leads to ST elevated myocardial infarction (STEMI), whereas partial occlusion leads to non-ST elevated myocardial infarction (NSTEMI) and unstable angina.
- Ischaemic damage can lead to left ventricular failure, arrhythmias, myocardial necrosis and rupture and pulmonary oedema.

Epidemiology

- IHD is the biggest cause of mortality in the Western world.
- Almost 150 000 people die of myocardial infarction each year in the UK.

Risk factors are classified as modifiable and non-modifiable:

- non-modifiable risk factors:
  - age
  - male sex
  - family history
  - race
  - socioeconomic status
- modifiable risk factors:
  - smoking
  - diabetes mellitus
  - hypercholesterolaemia
  - hypertension
  - obesity
  - sedentary lifestyle
  - diet.

- IHD is more common in males, although it becomes more frequent in females after the menopause.
- Those of South-East Asian background have a higher incidence of IHD than Whites.
- The incidence of IHD is far greater in those of low socioeconomic status than those of high status.

Tip

Although, a diet containing fresh fruit and vegetables is advocated in those at risk of IHD, clinical trials of pharmacological doses of antioxidants have failed to demonstrate any benefit at preventing IHD.

Signs and symptoms

The initial symptom in all types of IHD is a prolonged 'crushing' chest pain. This radiates from the centre of the chest towards the jaw, neck and arms. Some patients, especially the elderly, may experience a silent myocardial infarction, without any of the classical signs or symptoms. Other symptoms include:

- breathlessness
- collapse
- anxiety
- nausea/vomiting.

Signs of IHD include:

- pallor and sweating
- tachycardia or bradycardia, from either sympathetic or vagal activation
- hypotension

- oliguria
- cold extremities
- narrow pulse pressure
- lung crepitations.

Investigations

- Initial investigations centre on the use of ECG and the measurement of markers of myocardial damage.
- An elevation in the ST segment of the ECG leads to a diagnosis of STEMI and rapid treatment is necessary (Figure 5.1). Those without the change are termed as having either NSTEMI or unstable angina.

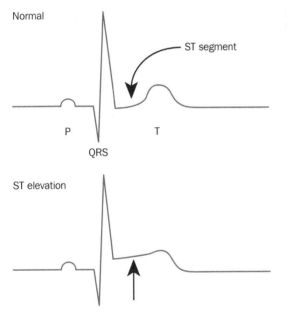

Figure 5.1 ECG showing normal trace and ST elevation.

- Ischaemia releases the protein troponin from cardiac monocytes. It is a highly sensitive marker of myocardial damage. As damage is progressive, it is recommended to test for the presence of the enzyme 12 h after the initial onset.
- Two forms of troponin may be measured, T or I. A myocardial infarction is indicated by serum troponin T of 0.1 ng/mL or serum troponin I of 1 ng/mL.
- Levels of troponin T of 0.01–0.1 ng/mL or troponin I of 0.1–1.0 ng/mL indicate some ischaemia but not myocardial infarction and this is termed unstable angina.

- Other tests performed would include a physical examination, focusing on the heart and lungs to determine any other pathologies, thyroid function tests, a diabetes screen, full blood count and urea and electrolytes.

Management

The management of IHD is rapidly evolving and comprises two phases: management of the acute phase and secondary prevention of further events.

Initial management

A diagnosis of the type of IHD event is often not possible until admission to hospital; therefore, initial management of all patients consists of:
- oxygen to reduce hypoxia
- aspirin 300 mg to reduce further thrombus formation
- glyceryl trinitrate to reduce ischaemia and associated chest pain
- IV morphine or diamorphine for pain relief
- metoclopramide for nausea.

In patients with STEMI, reperfusion of the ischaemic area is of utmost importance. This is achieved through either thrombolytic medication or interventional techniques.
- Thrombolytic medications include streptokinase and the tissue plasminogen activators, such as alteplase and tenecteplase. These act by aiding in the dissolution of the thromboembolism.
- The thrombolytic drugs are administered via IV injections or infusions and have been shown to achieve full reperfusion in up to 60% of patients.
- Contraindications to their use include:
  - active bleeding
  - high risk of bleeding, e.g. over 75 years of age
  - coagulation disorders
  - severe hypertension
  - history of haemorrhagic stroke
  - pregnancy
  - major surgery or trauma within the last 3 months
  - previously received streptokinase, so cannot receive it again because of antibody development at initial use.
- Percutaneous coronary intervention (PCI) is also used, especially in those for whom thrombolytic medications are contraindicated.
- PCI involves the use of peripherally inserted catheters to open occluded vessel(s) with a balloon, termed angioplasty. Metal stents may also be used to maintain the patency of the vessel (see Figure 3.1).

- Full platelet inhibition must be achieved prior to PCI, using clopidogrel 300–600 mg stat and glycoprotein IIb/IIIa inhibitors such as abciximab.

Secondary management

Secondary prevention of IHD after STEMI is attempted through use of a number of medications.

- *Lipid-lowering agents* should be prescribed for all patients, irrespective of their blood lipid levels. These should be at doses shown to be of benefit in IHD, e.g. simvastatin 40 mg daily.
- *Beta-blockers* should be initiated as soon as the patient is clinically stable. Bisoprolol and carvedilol are licensed for this indication in the UK. They should be initiated at a low dose and titrated up to the highest dose that is tolerated.
- *ACE inhibitors* should be started 24–48 h after myocardial infarction once the patient is clinically stable. Again, they should be started at a low dose and increased to the maximum tolerated dose.
- *Aldosterone antagonists* should be initiated in all those with signs or symptoms suggestive of left ventricular failure within 3 to 14 days after their myocardial infarction. Although spironolactone is the most widely used drug in this class, it is unlicensed for this indication. Eplerenone is licensed in the UK for this indication.

Those diagnosed with NSTEMI or unstable angina are at less immediate danger of death for their event; they are, however, at an increased risk of death in the months following the event. Management varies according to risk factors and severity of the episode.

- All patients receive dual antiplatelet therapy of aspirin 75 mg daily and clopidogrel 75 mg. Loading doses of 300 mg of each are administered on presentation.
- Aspirin is usually continued lifelong, unless there is a contraindication.
- It is recommended by NICE that clopidogrel is continued for 12 months after the episode.
- Unfractionated heparin infusions or low-molecular-weight heparins are used for 2 to 8 days after the onset of symptoms to prevent further thrombosis.
- Low-molecular-weight heparins, such as enoxaparin 1 mg/kg twice daily via subcutaneous injection, are the favoured treatment of choice as there are no intensive monitoring requirements and administration is simple.
- Anti-anginal drugs should be given to ease chest pain. Isosorbide mononitrate, beta-blockers or calcium-channel blockers (e.g. diltiazem or amlodipine) are commonly used.

Tip

Patients and their GPs are often unclear how long clopidogrel therapy is continued. For this reason, a 'clopidogrel card' has been developed and is given to patients after drug initiation at a number of hospitals.

Monitoring parameters

- Patients undergoing treatment for acute coronary syndromes receive a number of medications that affect clotting: antiplatelets, heparin, thrombolytic drugs and glycoprotein IIb/IIIa inhibitors. Therefore, patients should have clotting factors and full blood counts assessed at baseline and during treatment and should be monitored for signs of bleeding.
- Patients at high risk of bleeding when receiving two antiplatelet drugs may benefit from the addition of a proton pump inhibitor.
- Those started on ACE inhibitors and aldosterone antagonists need their serum creatinine and potassium assessed at baseline and 2 weeks after initiation because of the risk of hyperkalaemia and renal failure with these drugs.
- Patients should be regularly reviewed to ensure that dosage of beta-blocker and ACE inhibitor are titrated to the maximum tolerated. Dose-limiting effects may be a decrease in blood pressure, bradycardia with beta-blockers or renal impairment with ACE inhibitors.
- Liver function tests should be performed at baseline, 3 months and annually for those taking statins to ensure that the drugs do not cause hepatotoxicy. Patients should also be told to report any signs of liver damage.
- The presence of risk factors should be assessed and steps taken to modify those who are present, for example smoking cessation, appropriate exercise and dietary modification.
- Patients should be monitored for signs and symptoms of left ventricular function and arrhythmias after myocardial infarction, using ECG, echocardiograms and physical examination.

Tip

Pharmacists are well placed to advise patients on the need to continue their secondary prevention medications. This is important as patients often assume incorrectly that they do not need to continue them after the acute phase of their myocardial infarction.

Counselling

- Pharmacists can have a major role to play in the management of patients with IHD, especially in relation to the optimisation and monitoring of secondary prevention medication and minimising risk factors.
- All patients should be aware of the adverse effects and monitoring required for the medication.
- Patients need to be aware of the importance of continuing their medication for the

recommended time periods, which for the majority of the medications is lifelong.

- Reinforcement of lifestyle modifications, such as smoking cessation and diet, should be done where possible.
- Providing education on the signs of myocardial infarction to patients at high risk of event and the need for urgent medical attention can help to save their lives in the future.

Multiple choice questions

1. **Which of the following is *not* a sign or symptom of myocardial infarction?**
a. Crushing chest pain
b. Nausea
c. Hypertension
d. Breathlessness
e. Sweating

2. **Are the following statements true or false?**
a. All STEMI patients should receive an aldosterone antagonist once clinically stable.
b. Clopidogrel should be continued for 12 months after an episode of unstable angina.
c. When used for secondary prevention after a myocardial infarction, beta-blockers should be given at the lowest effective dose.
d. It is essential to monitor potassium levels in those receiving an ACE inhibitor and an aldosterone antagonist.
e. Patients can only receive one course of treatment with streptokinase in their lifetime.

Useful websites

www.nice.org.uk
www.bhf.org.uk

chapter 6
Stroke

Overview

- There are two main types of stroke: ischaemic and haemorrhagic. Ischaemic is the most common.
- Thrombolytic drugs are used to reduce the size of clots responsible for ischaemic stroke and must be given within 3 h of symptom onset.
- The management of haemorrhagic stroke mainly involves supportive care and the reversal of any underlying clotting abnormalities.
- Secondary prevention of ischaemic stroke involves the long-term use of antiplatelet drugs and the reduction of risk factors such as hypertension and diabetes.

Aetiology

- Approximately 85% of strokes are ischaemic and 15% haemorrhagic.
- Ischaemic strokes occur when there is blockage to one of the arteries carrying blood to the brain.
- Blockage may be from cerebral thrombosis, where the clot forms in a main artery to the brain, or cerebral embolism, where the clot forms elsewhere in the body before all or part of it is transported to the brain.
- A lacunar stroke may also occur, with clots in the small vessels within the brain.
- The lack of an adequate supply of oxygenated blood leads to the formation of areas of ischaemia within the brain.
- A haemorrhagic stroke occurs when there is bleeding from the vessels within the brain (intracranial) or the vessels on the surface of the brain into the space between the skull and the brain (subarachnoid).
- The area of brain that is damaged and the extent of the injury will determine the effect of the stroke on the patient.
- The left half of the brain controls the right side of the body and vice versa.
- The left half of the brain is also responsible for language production and understanding, whereas the right side is responsible for perceptual and spatial skills.
- A transient ischaemic attack (TIA) is defined as stroke symptoms that resolve within 24 h.
- Those suffering from a TIA are at a hugely increased risk of suffering a stroke.

Epidemiology

- Stroke is the most common cause of disability in UK adults.
- There are approximately 450 000 people living with a severe disability caused by stroke in the UK.
- Approximately 150 000 people have a stroke in the UK each year. It is the third leading cause of death in the UK, causing 60 000 deaths per year.
- The incidence of stroke rises with age but 1000 people under 30 suffer a stroke each year.
- There is an increased risk of stroke with decreasing socioeconomic status.
- People of Afro-Caribbean origin are twice as likely as Whites to suffer a stroke.
- Each patient that suffers a stroke costs the NHS over £15 000 in direct care costs in the 5 years following the event.

Risk factors for stroke include:

- smoking
- obesity
- high blood pressure
- diabetes
- sedentary lifestyle
- excessive alcohol intake
- atrial fibrillation
- male gender
- race.

Signs and symptoms

The signs and symptoms of stroke have a rapid onset and include:

- weakness, numbness or paralysis on one side of the body
- slurred speech or difficulty in finding words
- difficulty in understanding speech
- sudden blurred vision or blindness in one or both eyes
- confusion
- unsteadiness
- severe headache.

Weakness or paralysis may be manifest as drooping limbs or eyelids or dribbling mouth.

The signs of a TIA are identical to those of stroke but resolve within a few minutes or hours.

Investigations

- Investigations are required to determine where the stroke is, how serious it is and what has caused it.
- The priority is usually to determine the type of stroke suffered, so that appropriate initial therapy can be administered in a timely manner.
- This is achieved through the use of computed axial tomography (CT) or magnetic resonance imaging (MRI) of the brain. This will establish the type of stroke and the size and location of any haemorrhage or infarct.
- These assessments should be performed as soon as possible, ideally within the first few hours of the onset of symptoms.
- Further tests are done to establish risk factors for the stroke event, such as blood pressure to test for hypertension, blood and urinary glucose to test for diabetes and ECG to test for the presence of arrhythmias.
- A chest radiograph may be performed to assess the presence of any underlying heart or lung problems.
- Full blood counts, clotting screen and urea and electrolytes will determine any clotting disorders or liver or renal dysfunction that may have contributed to the stroke or may affect its treatment.
- A swallowing test will be performed as early as possible. This determines whether the patient's ability to swallow liquids and solids safely is impaired. Such impairment could lead to problems eating, drinking and taking medications. This could result in dehydration or aspiration of ingested items into the lungs.
- A type of ultrasound, a carotid Doppler, can be used to determine whether there is any restriction to the blood flow through the carotid arteries in the neck that supply the brain.

Management

Initial management is dependent on the type of stroke.

Ischaemic stroke
- An attempt to break down the clot using thrombolytic medication has become standard care in ischaemic stroke in recent years.
- Clot dissolution is attempted using alteplase at a dose of 0.9 mg/kg, with 10% of the dose given as a bolus injection and the remainder as an infusion over 1 h.
- Alteplase is only indicated for use within the first 3 h after symptom onset and must only be used by specialists trained in its use and in

patients who have had brain imaging to confirm that their stroke is ischaemic in nature.

- Homeostasis should be maintained through:
- administration of oxygen if required to maintain saturations above 95%
- blood sugars maintained between 4 and 11 mmol/L using insulin and glucose, especially in diabetic patients
- blood pressure kept below 185/110 mmHg for those who are candidates for thrombolytic therapy
- antihypertensive drugs should only be given to other patients where there is a hypertensive emergency.
- Antiplatelet therapy should be initiated within 48 h of onset. This is usually aspirin at a dose of 300 mg daily for 14 days, reduced to 75–150 mg daily lifelong. Clopidogrel may be used in those with known aspirin intolerance.

Haemorrhagic stroke

- These are no specific drug treatments for the management of haemorrhagic stroke.
- If the patient was taking warfarin, then a decision must be taken on whether to reverse the effects using IV vitamin K and prothrombin complex concentrate. In the majority of patients, the benefits of warfarin reversal will outweigh the risks.
- Supportive care is the same as that provided to those with ischaemic stroke, to maintain homeostasis and to ensure the patient is comfortable, hydrated and pain free.
- In some cases of primary intracranial haemorrhage, surgery may be appropriate especially if the patient has hydrocephalus and was previously fit.

Secondary prevention

- Those who have experienced an ischaemic stroke have an increased risk of a further stroke so secondary prevention is important.
- Antiplatelets are administered. Dypiridamole 200 mg modified-release capsules twice daily has been shown to decrease the risk of further strokes, but it is associated with an increased risk of life-threatening bleeds.
- Anticoagulation therapy with warfarin is more effective than antiplatelet drugs for preventing further episodes of stroke in those with atrial fibrillation.
- Attempts to correct risk factors should be made. This would include control of hypertension, hyperlipidaemia and diabetes, as well as diet modification, smoking cessation, limiting alcohol consumption and increasing exercise.

Transient ischaemic attack

- Those experiencing a TIA should be initiated on aspirin 300 mg daily, reducing to 75 mg daily after 14 days.
- They should be reviewed by a specialist and receive investigations including brain imaging if necessary. This should be done within 24 h if at high risk of further event or within 1 week if at low risk.
- An attempt to modify any risk factors should also be made.

> ## Tip
> Although statins are useful at reducing the risk of further events in those with hypercholesterolaemia, it is recommended that statins are not initiated within 48 h of stroke as there is a lack of evidence of benefit and safety if started in this time period.

Monitoring parameters

- Patients should be closely monitored to ensure they are well hydrated, free of pain and haemodynamically stable. This is done by monitoring urea and electrolytes, fluid balance, blood pressure, heart rate, blood glucose levels and temperature.
- Thrombolytics are associated with an increased risk of internal bleeding so should be avoided in those with significant risk factors such as recent surgery or trauma or underlying clotting abnormalities.
- The risk of bleeding is also increased in those who have received aspirin or other antiplatelet drugs.
- Antiplatelet drugs can also cause hypotension and increased temperature.
- In the long term, patients should have their risk factors monitored, such as diabetes, hypertension and blood lipids.
- Patients receiving long-term antiplatelet therapy should be monitored for signs of gastric bleeding and other intolerances.
- In patients receiving warfarin, the usual extensive monitoring of the international normalised ratio (INR) should be undertaken.

> ## Tip
> Many healthcare professionals are involved in the care of stroke patients. These include pharmacists, doctors, nurses, radiographers, speech and language therapists, dieticians, physiotherapists, occupational therapists and clinical psychologists. Each professional should be aware of the roles that each profession plays in the provision of patient care.

Counselling

- Patients and their carers should be aware of the risks of further strokes occurring. Knowledge of the signs and symptoms is important.
- Patients are assessed by speech and language therapists to determine whether their swallowing is impaired. If it is, an assessment should be made to determine any medication administration issues. Any that become apparent should be addressed as soon as possible.

Tip

Many stroke patients experience difficulty with swallowing, including an inability to swallow tablets and capsules. In these patients medications may have to be converted to liquid preparations, either proprietary or extemporaneous. In some cases, it may be necessary to change from one drug to another with similar activity in order to make administration possible.

- Patients should be fully educated regarding the importance of any medication they are taking to prevent a further stroke. They should have understanding of dosing, adverse effects and the likely duration of therapy.
- Those who have experienced a haemorrhagic stroke should know that this could affect future treatment of other conditions and that they should inform medical practitioners of it in the future.
- Patients should receive comprehensive and repeated guidance on how to reduce the risk of further episodes of ischaemic stroke by managing and reducing their risk factors.

Multiple choice questions

1. **Which of the following is not a common sign or symptom of stroke?**
a. Headache
b. Unilateral weakness
c. Blurred vision
d. Gradually deteriorating confusion
e. Slurred speech

2. **Are the following statements true or false?**
a. Alteplase is used in the treatment of haemorrhagic stroke.
b. Hypertensive patients should have their blood pressure tightly controlled in the acute phase of stroke.
c. Dypiridamole is normally used as an alternative to aspirin in the secondary prevention of stroke.
d. After ischaemic stroke, patients should receive lifelong aspirin unless there is intolerance or contraindication.
e. Alteplase is given up to 24 h after initial symptoms.

Useful websites

www.nice.org.uk
www.stroke.org.uk

The respiratory system

chapter 7
Asthma

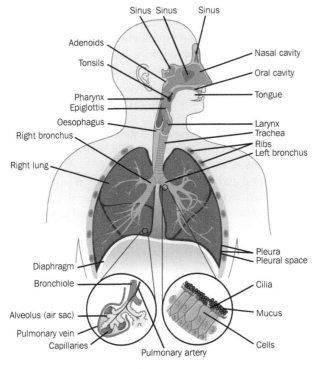

Figure 7.1 The respiratory system.

Overview

- Asthma is a chronic condition with a pattern of acute episodes separated by periods with few symptoms.
- It is managed using a stepwise approach.
- Management is mainly through the use of inhaled therapies.
- Patients can have a significant role in self-management.
- Ensuring patients know how to use their inhaler devices appropriately is a key factor in management.
- Acute episodes are potentially life-threatening events.

Tip

Although NSAIDs are generally considered to be contraindicated in asthmatic patients, a carefully taken drug history can often reveal that patients have taken over-the-counter preparations containing NSAIDs without any problem.

Aetiology

- The disease process results from hypersensitivity of the lungs to one or more stimuli (Table 7.1).
- The body reacts to stimuli to produce chronic bronchoconstriction.
- Allergens act on macrophages, T-lymphocytes, epithelial cells and eosinophils. Each produces inflammation through direct or neural mechanisms.
- Mast cells release histamine, leukotrienes and prostaglandins to induce bronchospasm.
- The immune response leads to marked hypertrophy and hyperplasia of bronchial smooth muscle, resulting in narrowing of the small airways.
- Bronchial gland and goblet cell hypertrophy results in excessive mucus production, often more viscous than usual. This can plug the airways in conjunction with epithelial and inflammatory cell debris.
- Airways become oedematous and mucociliary clearance is decreased.
- In the long term, the airways can become more responsive to triggers and acute bronchoconstriction can occur, leading to acute severe episodes.

Table 7.1 Common triggers in asthmatic patients

Trigger type	Examples
Allergens	Pollen, house dust mites, moulds, pets
Chemicals	Paints, cleaning products, aerosols, aluminium
Foods	Dairy products, food dyes, nuts, seafood
Industrial	Wood dust, colophony, cotton, smoke, sulphur dioxide
Medications	NSAIDs, beta-blockers
Others	Stress, exercise, cold air, viral infections, emotions

Epidemiology

- Prevalence is difficult to determine as there is an overlap with other respiratory conditions, such as chronic obstructive pulmonary disease (COPD), difficulty in diagnosis in children and variation in the classification of airway restriction.
- It is thought that there are 5.2 million people in the UK being treated for asthma, of whom 1.1 million are children.

- It is estimated that one in five households in the UK has a person suffering from asthma.
- Prevalence in children is thought to be approximately 5–10%, with 30–70% becoming asymptomatic by adulthood.
- Asthma is vastly more prevalent in the developed world than in the developing world, owing to increased exposure to environmental triggers, diet and stress.

Signs and symptoms

Patients can present with a range of symptoms; however, certain characteristics can help to diagnose, or exclude, asthma. Patients often describe fluctuating severity of symptoms, with varying time periods that may be symptom free. The most common symptoms indicative of asthma are:

- wheeze
- breathlessness
- chest tightness
- chronic cough.

Patients also have a history of atopic disorders such as eczema, family history of asthma or atopy, unexplained peripheral blood eosinophilia and widespread wheeze of auscultation of chest.

Symptoms and factors that may indicate an alternative disease state include a significant smoking history (i.e. greater than 20 pack-years), symptoms only with viral infections, voice disturbance, normal chest examination when symptomatic, dizziness, chronic productive cough in absence of wheeze and breathlessness.

Investigations

Initial diagnosis is made using the presence of clinical signs and symptoms but requires further tests to confirm.

Lung function tests

- A spirometer is used to determine the patient's forced expiratory volume in 1 s (FEV_1) and forced vital capacity (FVC). FEV_1 is a measure of the volume of air expelled in the first second of breathing out. FVC is a measure of the maximum volume of air it is possible for the patient to breathe out after taking maximal inspiration.
- The FEV_1/FVC ratio is used to determine the severity of airway obstruction. A patient with normal airways should have a value of approximately 0.75. In asthmatic patients, it is usually 0.7.
- Peak expiratory flow rate (PEFR) can be measured by the patient using a peak flow meter.
- Variability in readings of greater than 20% and at least 60 mL on 3 days of a week is highly suggestive of asthma.

- A peak flow meter can also allow patients to monitor their condition on a daily basis, particularly when they feel an increase in their symptoms.

Management

The management of asthma is split into two phases, chronic and acute. Acute asthma is an emergency.

Chronic management

The aim of treatment in the chronic phase is to control the disease. Control is defined as:

- no daytime symptoms
- no acute episodes
- no night-time awakening
- no need of rescue medication
- no limitations on activity owing to asthma
- normal lung function, defined as FEV_1 and/or PEFR 80% predicted or best
- minimal adverse effects.

A stepwise approach is utilised in the chronic management of asthma. There are five steps to therapy and treatment should be initiated at the most appropriate step for the patient's symptoms (Table 7.2).

- Treatment should be reviewed regularly and stepped up if control is inadequate or down if control is good.
- Patients should also be educated to avoid their known trigger factors where possible.
- The majority of treatments are administered via inhalation in order to minimise side-effects and maximise delivery to the target site.
- Patient's inhaler technique should be assessed at every review and counselling to improve should be provided or a change to the inhaler device considered if technique is not adequate.
- All asthmatic patients should receive 'reliever' inhalers for the relief of symptoms and those with steps 2 to 5 (Table 7.2) should receive 'preventer' inhalers.

Reliever medication

- *Beta-adrenoceptor agonists* are the basis of asthma therapy. Examples are salbutamol and terbutaline.
- They act on β_2-adrenoceptors to produce bronchodilation. They have some effect on β_2-adrenoceptors in cardiac tissue to produce tachycardia.
- Inhaled anticholinergic agents (e.g. ipratropium) have a slower onset but longer duration of action than the β_2-adrenoceptor agonist.

Table 7.2 Treatment steps in the chronic management of asthma in adults[a]

	Treatment
Step 1	Occasion relief with bronchodilator Inhaled short-acting β_2-agonist, e.g. salbutamol, when required Move to step 2 if required more than twice weekly, significant night time symptoms once weekly, or exacerbation within last 2 years requiring systemic steroids or nebulised bronchodilators
Step 2	Inhaled short-acting β_2-agonist when required Plus, standard dose inhaled corticosteroid regularly, e.g. beclometasone dipropionate 100–400 μg twice daily or equivalent
Step 3	Inhaled short-acting β_2-agonist when required Plus, standard dose inhaled corticosteroid regularly Plus, trial of inhaled long-acting β_2-agonist regularly, e.g. salmeterol or formeterol, to be stopped if no apparent benefit If asthma not controlled, ensure corticosteroid dose is at higher end of dose range and consider adding leukotriene receptor antagonist, theophylline or oral β_2-agonist
Step 4	Inhaled short-acting β_2-agonist when required Plus, high-dose inhaled corticosteroid regularly, e.g. beclometasone dipropionate 400–1000 μg twice daily or equivalent Plus, inhaled long-acting β_2-agonist regularly Plus, a 6 week trial of one or more of leukotriene receptor antagonist, theophylline or oral β_2-agonist
Step 5	Inhaled short-acting β_2-agonist when required Plus, high-dose inhaled corticosteroid regularly Plus, one or more long-acting bronchodilators Plus, regular oral prednisolone

[a]Patients can move up and down the steps as dictated by assessments.

- Inhaled anticholinergic agents are normally only used in acute severe asthma or in patients with mixed asthma and COPD.
- Inhaled *corticosteroids* are the most common agents used for the long-term control of asthma. The dose used should be the lowest effective dose for the patient and should be reviewed regularly.
- When corticosteroid dose reductions are felt to be appropriate, they should be done in increments of approximately 25–50% of the total dose every 3 months.
- Doses of inhaled corticosteroids are expressed as the equivalent dose of beclometasone given via CFC-containing metered dose inhaler (MDI). It is important to bear in mind the equivalence of the corticosteroid used to beclometasone when switching from one to another.
- Corticosteroids are usually initiated in patients who have had an exacerbation within the last 2 years while using inhaled β_2-adrenoceptor agonists three or more times per week, who have experienced symptoms three times a week, or who are awakened one night a week.
- Adrenal suppression is unlikely but is more likely to occur at doses of 2 mg per day.

- Inhaled corticosteroids can cause candidiasis and vocal harshness. This can be minimised with the use of large-volume spacer devices and rinsing the mouth after use.
- Long-acting β_2-adrenoceptor agonists (LABA) are added to patient's therapy when low-dose inhaled corticosteroids have had an inadequate response. Examples are salmeterol and formeterol.
- The long-acting β_2-adrenoceptor agonists should be trialed for 4 to 6 weeks and discontinued if there is no response.
- The long-acting β_2-adrenoceptor agonists are unsuitable as relievers and should not be used without inhaled corticosteroids.
- *Theophylline* or *aminophylline* are oral bronchodilators. They have a narrow therapeutic window, so patients require individual dosing regimens optimised using therapeutic drug monitoring.
- Toxicity with theophylline or aminophylline may present as vomiting, insomnia, fitting, arrhythmia, hyperglycaemia and hypotension.
- *Leukotriene antagonists*, such as montelukast, are oral agents useful for patients with difficulty in controlling asthma. They are especially useful in those with aspirin-induced asthma.
- Anti-IgE monoclonal antibodies are a new class of asthma treatment. The first agent in the class is omalizumab. Their use is restricted to those with severe persistent allergic asthma failing to respond to other agents. They are a very costly therapy and are currently rarely used.
- Long-term oral corticosteroids are only used in chronic management when other options have failed to adequately achieve treatment goals.
- Long courses of oral corticosteroids are associated with adrenal suppression, osteoporosis, skin thinning, peptic ulceration, bruising and many other adverse effects.
- In those requiring long-term oral steroids, agents such as oral gold, methotrexate and ciclosporin have been used with varying success. They should only be prescribed by specialists and their use must be closely monitored.

Tip

Salbutamol overdose is virtually impossible to achieve, so patients with acute severe asthma should use as much as they feel they require.

Acute management

Acute asthma is a life-threatening emergency. Patients should be reviewed and managed as soon as possible. The severity of the episode must be assessed and treated accordingly. It is classified into three types according to the results of the assessment:

- *moderate exacerbation*
- increasing symptoms

- PEFR 50–75% of best or predicted
- no features of acute severe asthma
- *acute severe asthma*: any one of PEFR 33–50% of best or predicted, respiratory rate 25 breaths/min, heart rate 110 beats/min or inability to complete sentences
- *life-threatening asthma*: the presence of any one of:
- PEFR 33% of best or predicted
- SpO_2 92% (peripheral oxygen saturation measured by pulse oximetry)
- PaO_2 8 kPa (arterial oxygen tension)
- normal $PaCO_2$ (arterial carbon dioxide tension)
- silent chest
- cyanosis
- feeble respiratory effort
- bradycardia, arrhythmia, hypotension
- exhaustion, confusion, coma.

Patients should be admitted if they have life-threatening asthma or acute severe asthma that fails to respond to initial treatment.

In those not requiring admission, treatment with increased doses of β_2-adrenoceptor agonists and a short course of corticosteroids (e.g. prednisolone 40–50 mg daily for 1 week) is normally sufficient.

In those requiring admission, further treatment is required.

- High-flow oxygen.
- Nebulised, high-dose β_2-adrenoceptor agonists.
- Nebulised ipratropium may be added if required.
- Oral corticosteroids, as above; IV hydrocortisone can be given in patients unable to tolerate oral therapy.
- A single dose of IV magnesium sulphate 1.2–2 g can be given to patients with acute severe asthma without a good response to inhaled bronchodilator therapy or with life-threatening asthma.
- IV aminophylline may be administered to those without adequate response to other therapies. It is given as an initial bolus of 250 µg, followed by an infusion of 500 µg/kg per hour. The bolus dose is omitted in those already taking aminophylline or theophylline therapy.
- Antibiotics are only necessary when there are clear clinical signs of infection.

Monitoring parameters

- Many patients can self-monitor their asthma using a peak flow meter and symptom diary.
- All patients should be reviewed by their medical team at appropriate intervals, at least

Tip

Inhalers are available in a wide range of devices. Pharmacists should be familiar with which drugs are available in each device and how each device is used.

annually for stable patients and more often for those with a history of acute severe episodes or inadequate control.

■ Patient's treatment should be stepped up and down whenever appropriate.
■ Monitoring should include an assessment of their symptoms, their objective lung function data and frequency of acute episodes.
■ The presence of any side-effects to drug therapy should be ascertained.

Counselling

■ Patients should have a firm knowledge of the actions and side-effects of the drugs they are taking.
■ The most appropriate inhaler devices should be utilised and patients should receive regular counselling on their use.
■ Patients should be told to seek prompt medical advice if there are any signs of acute severe asthma or gradual worsening of symptoms with a loss of response to inhaled β_2-adrenoceptor agonists.

Multiple choice questions

1. Which of the following is *not* a sign of asthma?
a. Shortness of breath
b. Chronic cough
c. Dizziness
d. Chest tightness
e. Wheeze

2. Are the following statements regarding asthma true or false?
a. Lung function tests are carried out to aid diagnosis.
b. There are six steps to asthma therapy.
c. Salbutamol is a beta-agonist.
d. Overdose with salbutamol is common in patients with asthma.

Useful websites

www.sign.ac.uk
www.brit-thoracic.org.uk
www.asthma.org.uk

chapter 8

Chronic obstructive pulmonary disease

Overview

- Chronic obstructive pulmonary disease is a progressive obstructive airway disease that causes significant morbidity and mortality.
- The main cause is smoking.
- Although there are some similarities with the pathology and medications used in asthma, the management of chronic obstructive pulmonary disease has some significant differences

Aetiology

- Chronic obstructive pulmonary disease (COPD) is the term used for the conditions that used to be described as chronic bronchitis and emphysema.
- The central and peripheral airways, lung parenchyma and vasculature are all affected in COPD.
- The most important process is chronic inflammation, although imbalances in proteinases and antiproteinases and oxidative stress also contribute.
- Inflammation occurs in the airways, parenchyma and vasculature.
- In the central airways, there is an increase in goblet cell proliferation, leading to excessive mucus production; ciliary dysfunction, leading to decreased clearance of mucus; and an increase in inflammatory cells.
- Bronchiolitis occurs in the peripheral airways in conjunction with an increase in inflammatory and goblet cells, resulting in fibrosis.
- In the parenchyma areas, such as the bronchioles and alveoli, there is a loss of elastin. This leads to a destruction of bronchioles and alveoli and airway collapse. This is termed emphysema.
- The walls of the pulmonary vasculature thicken through infiltration of inflammatory cells, leading to destruction of the vascular bed.

> **Tip**
>
> Airflow limitation in COPD has reversible and irreversible causes. The reversible causes are those mainly targeted by drug therapy. Reversible causes include bronchial accumulation of inflammatory cells and mucus, airway smooth muscle contraction and dynamic hyperinflation. Irreversible causes include airway fibrosis and narrowing and parenchymal destruction.

- Damage may be caused by overactivity of proteinases released by macrophages or neutrophils. Normally the antiproteinases, such as α_1-antitrypsin, inhibit the damage caused by these enzymes. Some individuals are deficient in this enzyme, while it is also deactivated by cigarette smoke.
- All of this damage leads to impaired gaseous exchange.
- COPD can also lead to systemic inflammation and muscle wasting, which contributes further to morbidity.

Epidemiology

Tip

As smoking is the largest risk factor for COPD, encouraging patients who continue to smoke to give up is the most important aspect of treatment.

- COPD is the fourth leading cause of mortality worldwide.
- Its management costs the NHS approximately half a billion pounds per year.
- It is the leading cause of lost working days in the UK.
- Its main cause is smoking; however, environmental and workplace pollution may also contribute. Incidence is highest in highly industrialised areas, particularly amongst those such as coal miners and foundry workers.
- It is more common in men than women, but this mainly reflects higher smoking rates amongst men.
- Approximately 600 million people worldwide are thought to have the disease, with the incidence increasing with greater industrialisation.
- Not all smokers develop COPD, so it is thought that genetics may play a part in determining who will develop the disease.

Signs and symptoms

The majority of patients will have all the main symptoms; however, the severity of each may differ. Symptoms include:
- exertional breathlessness
- chronic cough
- regular sputum production
- frequent winter 'bronchitis'
- wheeze
- a barrel chest, which may develop as the disease progresses.

Pulmonary hypertension can lead to jugular distension, hepatomegaly and peripheral oedema.

Measurement of breathlessness

Breathlessness is measured using the MRC dyspnoea scale:[1]

grade 1: not troubled by breathlessness except on strenuous exercise

grade 2: short of breath when hurrying or walking up a slight hill

grade 3: walks slower than contemporaries on level ground because of breathlessness, or has to stop when walking at own pace

grade 4: stops for breath after walking about 100 m or after a few minutes on level ground

grade 5: too breathless to leave the house, or breathless when dressing or undressing.

Investigations

■ Lung function tests are the key to diagnosis and should be performed in patients with a suspicion of COPD.

■ As with asthma, forced expiratory volume in 1 s (FEV_1) and forced vital capacity (FVC) are the key measurements taken during lung function tests.

■ Airway obstruction is defined as an FEV_1 80% of predicted for the patient and FEV_1/FVC ratio of 0.7.

■ Vital capacity (VC) decreases with bronchitis and emphysema.

■ Residual volume (RV) increases with both; however, it is usually increased more in emphysema.

■ Total lung volume increases in emphysema as more air remains trapped within the lung during respiration.

■ Smoking history should be determined, as should exposure to other potential risk factors, for example through occupation.

■ Other investigations include chest radiography to exclude other causes, full blood count, body mass index, α_1-antitrypsin status, chest CT if the spirometry results seem unexpected and ECG to assess whether the patient has cor pulmonale.

■ FEV_1 can be used to define the severity of COPD:

– mild: FEV_1 80–50% of predicted

– moderate: FEV_1 30–49% of predicted

– severe: FEV_1 less than 30% of predicted.

The key differences in clinical features of asthma and COPD are shown in Table 8.1.

Table 8.1 The key differences in clinical features of asthma and chronic obstructive pulmonary disease (COPD)

Clinical feature	COPD	Asthma
Smoker or ex-smoker	Nearly all	Possibility
Symptoms present before 35 years of age	Rare	Common
Chronic productive cough	Common	Uncommon
Breathlessness	Persistent and progressive	Variable
Night-time waking from breathlessness and/or wheeze	Uncommon	Common
Significant diurnal or day-to-day variability of symptoms	Uncommon	Common

Management

- The aim of treatment is to:
- – prevent disease progression
- – provide symptomatic relief
- – prevent and treat complications and exacerbations
- – improve exercise tolerance.
- As with asthma, patients receive the majority of their medication via inhalation, either with inhaler devices or nebulisers.

Chronic management

- The chronic management of COPD follows a stepwise approach.
- Initial therapy is with short-acting bronchodilators, either β_2-adrenoceptor agonists or anticholergic drugs.
- These are given on an as required basis for the relief of symptoms.
- If they are ineffective, combining an agent from each class may be effective.
- In patients that remain symptomatic, a long-acting bronchodilator should be added. This could again be either a β_2-agonist, such as salmeterol or formeterol, or the anticholinergic tiotropium.
- Inhaled corticosteroids, such as beclometasone, budesonide and fluticasone, are indicated in those with moderate or severe COPD, or those with mild disease who experienced at least two exacerbations in the preceding 12 months.
- Oral theophyllines may be trialed in those who remain symptomatic.
- Patients with COPD may require high doses of bronchodilators, which may be administered via inhalers or nebulisers.
- There is little evidence that administering corticosteroids via nebulisation provides any addition benefit over the inhaled route, but it is associated with more adverse effects.
- Some patients may require oxygen therapy at home. In those requiring long-term oxygen it must be used for at least 15 h per day to provide optimal benefit.

Tip

Combination inhalers featuring fixed doses of a corticosteroid and a long-acting β_2-agonist are available in a number of inhaler device forms and may be useful in improving compliance in those on stable doses of the individual components. Care must be taken that the patient does not continue to use separate inhalers in addition.

Acute exacerbations

- Acute exacerbations are associated with increased morbidity and mortality.
- Acute exacerbations are characterised by an increase in dyspnoea, sputum purulence and sputum volume.
- Initial management involves:
- – an increase in the use of short-acting bronchodilators, via the nebulised route if inhalation fails to produce an adequate effect

- oral corticosteroids, e.g. prednisolone 30 mg daily for 7–14 days
- antibiotics where there are clear signs of infection, such as purulent sputum
- antibiotics used should be active against the most common causative bacteria, *Haemophylus influenzae*, *Streptococcus pneumoniae* and *Moraxella catarrhalis*; amoxicillin, doxycycline and clarithromycin are commonly used
- oxygen may be needed to keep oxygen saturation 90%
- IV theophylline may be utilised in those failing to respond to inhaled bronchodilators.

Monitoring parameters

- All patients with COPD should be reviewed at least annually. Those with stable disease can be managed in primary care but those with unstable or rapidly deteriorating disease (e.g. a decrease in FEV_1 of 500 mL in 5 years) should be under the care of a specialist.

  Tip

  Pneumococcal vaccination and annual influenza vaccination are recommended for all with COPD, regardless of the severity of their disease.

- At each review, patients should have their lung function, body mass index (BMI) and MRC dyspnoea score checked to provide an objective measure of disease.
- Subjective measurements should also include symptoms, presence of long-term complication, frequency of exacerbations, inhaler technique, depression and the need for further treatment.
- Subjective and objective measurements can often lead to differing conclusions regarding the state of the patient's disease so both must be assessed.
- The current smoking status of patient should be assessed using open questions, and those continuing to smoke should be encouraged to quit, with referral to local services provided.
- Patients' understanding of their condition and their medication should be assessed and any necessary education provided.
- Patients should be aware of potential side-effects of their medicines and the need to report those that are potentially troublesome and serious, such as candidiasis with corticosteroids and toxicity with theophylline.

Counselling

- Pharmacists can provide important support to patients with COPD by ensuring that patients understand their disease and medications.
- Inhaler technique is inadequate in patients with COPD (and asthma) and all patients should receive regular counselling on how

to use their devices. Even patients who previously demonstrated good technique have been shown to have poor technique when reassessed at a later date.

■ Patients should be made aware of the signs of an acute exacerbation. In those with frequent exacerbations and a good understanding of their disease, it may be possible for them to self-treat minor exacerbations using emergency courses of steroids and antibiotics.

Multiple choice questions

1. Which of the following are characteristics of COPD?
a. Significant smoking history
b. Chronic productive cough
c. Day to day variation in symptoms
d. Overactivity of α_1-antitrypsin
e. Breathlessness

2. Are the following statements regarding treatment of COPD true or false?
a. Prevents disease progression.
b. Provides symptomatic relief.
c. Prevents and treats complications and exacerbations.
d. Improves exercise tolerance.

Reference

1. Fletcher CM *et al.* (1959). The significance of respiratory symptoms and the diagnosis of chronic bronchitis in a working population *Br Med J* 2:257–266.

Useful websites

http://www.lunguk.org/
www.brit-thoracic.org.uk
www.nice.org.uk

Gastrointestinal
system

chapter 9
Inflammatory bowel disease

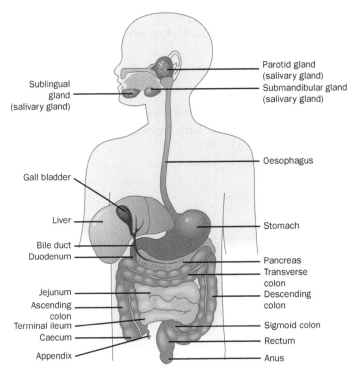

Figure 9.1 The gastrointestinal tract.

Sublingual gland (salivary gland)

Parotid gland (salivary gland)

Submandibular gland (salivary gland)

Oesophagus

Gall bladder

Liver

Stomach

Bile duct

Duodenum

Pancreas

Transverse colon

Jejunum

Descending colon

Ascending colon

Terminal ileum

Sigmoid colon

Caecum

Rectum

Appendix

Anus

Overview

- Inflammatory bowel disease can be classed as Crohn's disease and ulcerative colitis.
- Ulcerative colitis affects the large bowel only, Crohn's disease affects any part of the GI tract.
- Treatment aims are to induce and maintain remission and prevent secondary complications.
- Inflammation is controlled with aminosalicylates and corticosteroids.
- Immunosuppressants (cytokine inhibitors) are used in severe or refractory disease.

Aetiology

The aetiology of inflammatory bowel disease (IBD) is not known. Factors affecting the condition include:

- diet, e.g. fat intake, refined carbohydrates
- smoking: increases risk of relapse
- drugs, e.g. NSAIDs aggravate IBD
- stress: triggers the condition
- genetic: IBD is hereditary and is common in relatives of patients
- intestinal microflora: developed tolerance to microflora.

IBD can be divided into ulcerative colitis (UC), affecting the large bowel only, and Crohn's disease (CD), affecting any part of the GI tract from mouth to anus.

Epidemiology

- There are 6 new cases per 100 000 yearly.
- IBD is present worldwide, with prevalence in Western cultures.
- Jews are more prone to IBD.
- CD is more common in females.

Signs and symptoms

Crohn's disease:
- abdominal pain
- diarrhoea
- weight loss
- malaise
- vomiting
- anorexia.

Ulcerative colitis:
- diarrhoea with blood and mucus (passing up to 10–20 watery stools daily)
- lower abdominal pain
- lethargy
- anorexia.

Investigations

Tip

p-ANCA is usually positive in UC and negative in CD.

- Blood tests can detect anaemia, iron and folate deficiency, low serum vitamin B_{12}, raised erythrocyte sedimentation rate (ESR) and C-reactive protein (CRP), raised white cell count, p-ANCA (perinuclear-staining antineutrophil cytoplasmic antibody), blood cultures, liver enzymes.

- Stool cultures are taken when diarrhoea is present.
- Imaging includes radiography and MRI.
- Colonoscopy is useful in UC.

Management

The aim of treatment is to:
- control symptoms
- maintain remission
- induce remission
- avoid secondary complications.

Treatment covers particular aspects of IBD.

Tip

Total parenteral nutrition (TPN) may be indicated for malnourished patients where enteral feeding is not adequate. In some cases, both enteral and parenteral feeding may be required.

- *Nutrition*: malabsorption leads to deficiencies in vitamins, minerals and electrolytes. These are corrected accordingly (e.g. multivitamins). Nutritional supplementation (e.g. ensure plus, complain) compensates for poor food intake.
- *Corticosteroids* (e.g. hydrocortisone, prednisolone) are effective in inducing remission. Liquid or foam enemas are of benefit in localised rectal disease; oral or parental formulations are used in severe or extensive disease.
- *Aminosalicylates* (e.g. sulfasalazine, olsalazine) have an active metabolite 5-aminosalicylic acid, which has inflammatory properties and can induce and maintain remission.
- *Immunosuppressants* (e.g. azathioprine, ciclosporin, methotrexate): azathioprine has steroid-sparing properties and so lower doses of steroids may be prescribed. Methotrexate is used in CD for inducing and maintaining remission. Ciclosporin is prescribed in refractory UC.
- *Cytokine inhibitors* (e.g. infliximab) are anti-inflammatory through their action in reducing proinflammatory cytokines. Inflixamab inhibits the binding of tumour necrosis factor.
- *Antibiotics* (e.g. metronidazole) are useful in CD but ineffective in UC.
- *Surgery*: most patients will eventually require surgery if medical treatment fails; it also elimates the risk of colorectal cancer developing.
- *Probiotics* contain live microorganisms or natural gut flora and can maintain remission.

Ulcerative colitis
- Rectal formulations are recommended if the disease is confined to the rectum or left side of the colon.
- Foam enemas treat inflammation up to 20 cm. Rectal aminosalicylates are more effective in inducing remission than rectal corticosteroids.
- Liquid enemas are effective to treat inflammation from 30–60 cm.

- Oral aminosalicylates are used in more severe disease. Mesalazine is unstable in an acidic environment and so is rapidly absorbed from the GI tract. Formulations have been prepared to minimise this breakdown, for example coating tablets with pH-dependent resin.
- Oral corticosteroids may be used to induce remission. If long-term corticosteroids are required, azathioprine may be co-prescribed as it has steroid-sparing effects, thus minimising steroid side-effects

Crohn's disease
- Corticosteroid therapy is used first-line in CD.
- Azathioprine is usually co-precribed, acting as a steroid sparer and aiding in withdrawal of the steroid once remission is maintained.
- NICE has issued guidelines on the use of infliximab in severe CD.

Tips

Budesonide is licensed for CD and offers fewer side-effects than prednisolone as it is rapidly metabolised by the first-pass effect.

If patients experience dose-related side-effects with an older aminosalicylate, a newer one such as mesalazine can be tried as they have fewer side-effects.

Monitoring parameters

- High doses of corticosteroids increase the risk of side-effects such as moon face, osteoporosis, hypertension, diabetes, mood disturbances, lack of sleep, cataracts and glaucoma; they also increase the risk of infections.
- Side-effects of the aminosalicylates include nausea, vomiting, rash, metallic taste, abdominal pain, haemolytic anaemia, agranulocytosis, peripheral neuropathy, yellow colour of body fluids and staining of soft contact lenses.
- Side-effects of azathioprine include flu-like symptoms, nausea and diarrhoea.
- Methotrexate can cause nausea, vomiting, abdominal pain, hepatotoxicity, bone marrow suppression, pneumonitis; *Dosing should be once weekly*.
- Ciclosporin side-effects include tremor, headache, gum hypertrophy, hirsutism, neurotoxicity, hepatotoxicity, hypertension and nephrotoxicity.
- Hypersensitivity reactions may occur with the cytokine inhibitors and immune responses are affected; patients require close monitoring.

Counselling

- Aminosalicylates may discolour the urine and body fluids and turn soft contact lenses yellow. The patient should be reassured that it is nothing to be alarmed about.
- Regular blood tests are required if the patient is taking immunosuppressants and aminosalicylates.
- Side-effects of each drug should be explained to the patient.
- Formulations should be explained, particularly if rectal administration is required.
- It is important that the patient is maintained on the same brand of aminosalicylate. The patient must be told to remind any healthcare professional of the brand they are taking.
- Patients should be counselled on how to monitor blood dyscrasias: fever, malaise, flu-like symptoms, sore throat. They must seek immediate medical advice if this occurs.
- Patients should not withdraw steroid treatment unless advised to do so by a healthcare professional.
- If nausea occurs with any of the drugs, it is best to take it with food.

Multiple choice questions

1. Are the following statements true or false?
a. UC can affect any part of the GI tract.
b. Cushinoid effect can be a side-effect of prednisolone.
c. Mesalazine is metabolised in the GI tract.
d. If a patient experiences a metallic taste in their mouth, they may have a blood dyscrasia.

2. Are the following statements regarding IBD true or false?
a. UC affects the large bowel only.
b. Treatment aims include inducing remission.
c. NSAIDs may aggravate IBD.
d. A colonoscopy may be of benefit in Crohn's disease.
e. Anorexia is a sign of IBD.

Useful websites

http://www.nhsdirect.nhs.uk
http://www.nice.org.uk

chapter 10

Gastro-oesophageal reflux disease

Overview

- Gastro-oesophageal reflux disease is associated with heartburn and difficulty in swallowing.
- Management includes lifestyle changes, antacids, histamine H_2 receptor antagonists and proton pump inhibitors.
- In some severe cases where drug treatment fails, surgery may be an option.

Aetiology

- Gastro-oesophageal reflux disease (GORD) occurs when the oesophageal mucosa is exposed to the gastric contents for prolonged episodes.
- Causes include:
- hiatus hernia
- abnormalities of the lower oesophageal sphincter
- lifestyle
- increased intra-abdominal pressure
- delayed gastric emptying
- delayed oesophageal clearance.

Signs and symptoms

- Belching
- Bloating
- Heartburn
- Regurgitation
- Chest pain
- Cough
- Upper abdominal discomfort.

Investigations

- Endoscopy is the investigation of choice if complications are suspected.
- Test for *Helicobacter pylori*.

Tips

Extensive symptom history and evaluation should be carried out before treating patients, especially in the elderly.

Young to middle-aged patients can be treated empirically if they present with typical GORD symptoms.

Management

- The aim of treatment is to manage symptoms.
- Lifestyle changes should be promoted (see Counselling).
- *Antacids* and *alginates* produce a raft over the oesophageal mucosa, thus protecting it. Some antacids have a low sodium content (1 mmol per tablet or 10 mL dose; BNF section 1.1 lists preparations with low sodium content). They may be of benefit to patients with hypertension or heart disease.
- *Histamine H_2 receptor antagonists* relieve symptoms by reducing acid secretion.
- *Proton pump inhibitors* (PPI) relieve symptoms by suppressing acid secretion through inhibition of the enzyme hydrogen–potassium adenosine triphosphatase (H^+–K^+ ATPase).
- A PPI is given at the highest tolerated dose for 4–6 weeks.
- A lower dosage of the PPI is given as maintenance and the patient should be reviewed.
- Some patients require lifelong therapy and are maintained at the lowest possible dose.

Tips

PPIs have a better symptom management profile for GORD than do the H_2 receptor antagonists.
   Metoclopramide (prokinetic) accelerates gastric emptying and can also be used to relieve GORD symptoms.

Counselling

- Life style changes such as weight loss and smoking cessation should be promoted.
- Elevating the bed head can help if symptoms present during the night.
- Tight clothes should be avoided.
- Certain foods, such as caffeine, citrus fruits, fizzy drinks, should be avoided.

Multiple choice questions

1. Which of the following preparations does *not* contain low sodium?
a. Alu-cap
b. Maalox
c. Magnesium trisilicate mixture BP
d. Asilone
e. Altacite Plus

2. Are the following statements regarding GORD true or false?
a. Citrus foods may aggravate GORD.
b. Metoclopramide may induce gastric emptying.

c.   Gastric bleeding is a symptom of GORD.
d.   MRI scan may be used to diagnose GORD.

Useful websites

http://www.refluxadvice.co.uk
http://www.nhsdirect.nhs.uk

chapter 11

Peptic ulcer disease

Overview

- The two main causes of peptic ulcers are *Helicobacter pylori* and NSAIDs.
- The disease can be diagnosed by endoscopy.
- Management of NSAID-induced ulcers involves discontinuing the NSAID and a protein pump inhibitor.
- Management of *H. pylori*-induced ulcers requires triple therapy eradication with antibiotics.
- Symptoms include bloating, bleeding and vomiting.

Aetiology

Damage to the small intestine or stomach results in a peptic or duodenal ulcer. Causes include:

- *Helicobacter pylori*: a bacterial protein activates the inflammatory cascade
- drugs: NSAIDs in particular, causing mucosal damage by inhibiting cyclo-oxygenase (responsible for prostaglandin production)
- smoking
- excessive alcohol consumption.

Tips

Enteric-coated NSAIDs may prevent superficial damage but do not reduce the risk of developing an ulcer. Ulcer prophylaxis is recommended for patients at risk of developing an ulcer (e.g. having long-term NSAID or steroid therapy).

Epidemiology

- Peptic ulcer disease affects all age groups.
- Those aged 65 years are most susceptible.
- *H. pylori*-induced peptic ulcers are usually seen in communities of low social class with basic living standards.

Signs and symptoms

- Abdominal pain 1–3 h after meals (pain relieved by food or antacids)
- Nausea
- Vomiting
- Dyspepsia
- Bloating and belching.

- If any of the following warning symptoms are present, patient should seek medical advice and may need endoscopy:
- pain on swallowing
- dysphagia
- weight loss
- GI bleed
- anaemia
- non-stop vomiting
- drug use such as anticoagulants or NSAIDs.

Investigations

- Endoscopy is the investigation of choice. Endoscopy is an expensive procedure and is usually carried out when patients presents with warning symptoms.
- Radiology is not as accurate as endoscopy.
- *H. pylori* can be detected by:
- urea breath test
- stool antigen test
- antibody testing.

Tip

PPIs are more effective than H_2 antagonists in:
- treatment of NSAID-induced ulcers when the NSAID is being continued
- prophylaxis of NSAID-induced ulcers.

Management

- *H. pylori*-induced ulcers: antibiotic triple therapy for 1 week.
- NSAID-associated ulcers: discontinue NSAID and treat with the following:
- histamine H_2 receptor antagonists
- proton pump inhibitors (PPI)
- prostaglandin analogue.

Histamine H_2 receptor antagonists
Examples are cimetidine and ranitidine.
- Drugs are histamine analogues.
- Histamine receptors are blocked in the parietal cells in the gastric mucosa, thus acid secretion is inhibited.
- They have little benefit in treatment and managment of peptic ulcer disease.
- Drugs are effective in NSAID-induced ulcers if the NSAID is discontinued.

Proton pump inhibitors
Examples are omeprazole and lansoprazole.
- Gastric acid secretion is dependent on hydrogen–potassium adenosine triphosphatase (H^+–K^+ ATPase).

- PPIs are inactive prodrugs that activate in the acidic environment of the proton pump and then bind irreversibily to the pump, inhibiting acid secretion.

Prostaglandin analogue

Example is misoprostol.
- Synthetic prostaglandin analogues have protective and antisecretory properties.
- They are used for prevention of NSAID-associated ulcers in the frail and elderly.

Triple therapy

Triple therapy for *H. pylori*-induced peptic ulcers is usually for a week and comprises two antibiotics and a PPI (Table 11.1). Regimens over 2 weeks have higher eradication rates but can lead to poor concordance and compliance, thus rendering the treatment ineffective.

NSAID-induced ulcers can also be *H. pylori* positive; patients, therefore, also need to be treated via triple therapy and the NSAID discontinued.

Table 11.1 Regimens for the eradication of *Helicobacter pylori* in adults: acid suppressant plus two antibiotics

Acid suppressant	Antibiotic (two used)		
	Amoxicillin	Clarithromycin	Metronidazole
Esomeprazole 20 mg twice daily	1 g twice daily	500 mg twice daily	–
	–	250 mg twice daily	400 mg twice daily
Lansoprazole 30 mg twice daily	1 g twice daily	500 mg twice daily	–
Omeprazole 20 mg twice daily	1 g twice daily	500 mg twice daily	–
	500 mg three times daily	–	400 mg three times daily
Rabeprazole 20 mg twice daily	1 g twice daily	500 mg twice daily	–
	–	25 mg twice daily	400 mg twice daily
Pantoprazole 40 mg twice daily	1 g twice daily	500 mg twice daily	–
	–	25 mg twice daily	400 mg twice daily

Adapted from *British National Formulary* 56.

Monitoring parameters

- Side-effects of PPIs include GI disturbances, headache, flatulence and abdominal pain.
- Side-effects of H_2 antagonists include GI disturbances, headache rash and tiredness.
- Side-effects of prostaglandin analogues include diarrhoea and abnormal vaginal bleeding; they should not be used in women of childbearing age unless the benefit outweighs risk.

Tips

- Patients should be monitored for efficacy of treatment using the urea breath test with or without an endoscopy.

Counselling

- Smoking delays ulcer healing.
- NSAIDs should be discontinued where possible; a cyclo-oxygenase antagonist (e.g. rofecoxcib) can be considered if appropriate.
- Patients should be cautioned when purchasing NSAIDS over the counter.
- Side-effects of the drugs should be explained.
- Patients taking medication for *H. pylori* infection should be advised on the importance of finishing the course.
- In some patients, abdominal pain may persist after therapy, but it subsides after a few days; over-the-counter antacids may help to relieve this symptom.
- PPIs prescribed for the prophylaxis of NSAID-induced ulcers should be continued and not stopped until next review.

Multiple choice questions

1. **Are the following statements true or false?**
a. *H. pylori* is a bacterium causing a peptic ulcer.
b. Belching is a symptom of peptic ulcer disease.
c. Misoprostol is safe to give in pregnancy.
d. *H. pylori* can be detected by radiography.

2. **Are the following statements regarding peptic ulcer disease true or false?**
a. Dysphagia is a warning symptom of gastro-oesophageal reflux disease.
b. *H. pylori* eradication is usually a 2 week course.
c. Prostaglandin analogues have antisecretory effects.
d. Histamine H$_2$ receptor antagonists have little value in the treatment of peptic ulcer disease.
e. *H. pylori* can be detected with the urea breath test.

Useful website

http://www.nhsdirect.nhs.uk

chapter 12

Constipation

Overview

- Constipation is defined as the passing of hard stools infrequently, twice a week or less.
- There are many causes of constipation, including medication and diseases.
- It can be treated without drug therapy, by improving diet, increasing fluid intake and increasing exercise.
- Bulk-forming laxatives, stimulant laxatives, faecal softeners and osmotic laxatives are used to treat constipation

Aetiology

- Constipation is the passing of hard stools less frequently than a person's normal bowel habit.
- It involves straining and can be accompanied by pain.
- Causes include:
- poor diet: low in fibre or fluid
- drugs: there are over 20 classes of drug that may cause constipation
- dehydration
- electrolyte disturbances, e.g. hypokalaemia
- immobility
- pregnancy
- diseases, e.g. colon cancer
- poor bowel habit
- laxative abuse.

Tips

An individual normally defecates between three times a day and once every two days.

Constipation is caused by many factors. In order to make an informed decision of the presence of this symptom and its treatment, a full history needs to be taken, including the type of stools, frequency and other symptoms associated with it.

Epidemiology

- Constipation affects all age groups.
- The elderly are most susceptible.
- There is a higher incidence of females reported as suffering with constipation.
- Formula-fed babies are more likely to have constipation than breast-fed babies.
- Over 700 medicinal products have constipation listed as a side-effect.

Signs and symptoms

- Mild abdominal discomfort
- Distension
- Hard stools
- Small stools.

Management

The aim of treatment is to retain normal bowel habit and produce softer stools.

Tips

Patients increasing fibre in their diet are also advised to increase their water intake to 2 L a day.

A high-fibre diet may not be suitable for constipation-induced by opioids.

Non-drug treatment

- Increase fluid intake
- Reduce caffeine
- Increase intake of fibre
- Exercise.

Drug treatment

There are four classes of drugs used to manage constipation. Liquid paraffin is not recommended for prescribing and is no longer used as a faecal softener in treating constipation today.

Bulking agents

Example is ispaghula.

- Bulking agents stimulate colonic mucosal receptors, promoting peristalsis.
- They are used when dietary fibre cannot be increased in a patient and hard stools are present.

Osmotic laxatives

Examples are lactulose and magnesium salts.

- Osmotic laxatives retain fluid in the bowel.
- They also change the water distribution in faeces to produce softer stools.

Stimulant laxatives

Example is senna bisacodyl.

- These stimulate colonic nerves and causes movement of the faecal mass.
- They reduce reabsorption of water.
- Stool production is stimulated within 8–12 h.

Lubricants and stool softeners

Example is docusate sodium

- These act by reducing surface tension and so increase the penetration of intestinal fluids into the faecal mass.
- They may have weak stimulant properties.

Laxatives are of value in drug-induced constipation.

Monitoring parameters

- Frequency of bowel movements should be monitored with all laxatives.
- Side-effects of bulking agents include flatulence and abdominal distension.
- Side-effects of osmotic laxatives include flatulence, cramps and abdominal discomfort.
- Side-effects of stimulant laxatives include abdominal cramp, diarrhoea and hypokalaemia.
- Side-effects of faecal softeners include abdominal cramps and diarrhoea.

Counselling

- Improving diet is of importance and eating foods rich and fibre and low in animal fats is of benefit.
- Increasing fluid intake will help to soften stools.
- Decrease caffeine intake as this can act as a diuretic and worsen the constipation.
- Exercise is recommended to help to relax and contract the abdominal muscles.
- Before prescribing laxatives, it is important to take a full history of the patient's condition.
- Patients taking bulk laxatives should be recommended to drink at least 2 L of water in 24 h.
- Patients taking stimulant laxatives should be informed that they may have their effect within 8–12 h; therefore, they are best taken at night. If a rapid response is required, a stimulant suppository, such as glycerin, may be given.
- If lactulose is prescribed, patients should be advised to take the medication regularly, as it takes 48 h before an effect is exerted.

Multiple choice questions

1. Which of the following is used to treat constipation?
a. Sodium docusate
b. Propranolol
c. Loperamide

d. Oral rehydration salts

e. Furosemide

2. Are the following statements true or false?

a. There is no value of exercise in constipation.

b. Lactulose can be taken on a when required basis.

c. Breast-fed babies do not suffer with constipation.

d. Glycerin is given as a suppository and has a rapid onset of action.

Useful website

http://www.nhsdirect.nhs.uk

chapter 13

Diarrhoea

Overview

- Diarrhoea is the passing of loose and watery stools.
- Causes include broad-spectrum antibiotics and certain types of bacteria including *Escherichia coli*.
- A full patient history is required as diarrhoea is a symptom not a disease and its root cause needs to be identified.
- Symptoms include abdominal cramps and vomiting.
- First-line treatment is to take plenty of fluids and oral rehydration salts.
- Drug treatment is rarely necessary; but drugs such as codeine phosphate and loperamide can be used to relieve the diarrhoea

Aetiology

Diarrhoea is not a disease in itself; it is a sign of an underlying problem that needs to be investigated.

- There is increased passing of loose or watery stools.
- Viral gastroenteritis is a common cause in children and is self-limiting.
- Identified causes include *Escherichia coli*, *Clostridium perfringens* and *Salmonella*, *Shigella* spp.
- Many drugs can cause diarrhoea.
- Antibiotics, especially broad-spectrum drugs, induce diarrhoea.

Tip

If bloody diarrhoea (dysentery) is present, an invasive organism, such as *Salmonella*, may be the likely cause and referral to the doctor is necessary.

Signs and symptoms

- Loose stools
- Watery stools
- Anorexia
- Nausea
- Vomiting
- Abdominal cramps
- Flatulence
- Bloating
- Dehydration.

Tip

It is important to take a full history in order to identify the cause of the diarrhoea. The record of onset of symptoms is of value as it can help to identify the underlying problem.

Dehydration is a common problem in diarrhoea, and the clinical signs should be assessed. These include:

- decreased skin turgor
- dizziness
- postural hypotension
- tiredness.

Investigations

- A full drug history should be taken before investigating the causative factor. This can help to eliminate drug-induced diarrhoea.
- Stool cultures are taken if dysentery is present or if the diarrhoea persists for more than 48 h.
- If severe symptoms are occurring, the patient requires hospitalisation or a broad-spectrum antibiotic is being taken, testing for *Clostridium difficile*-induced pseudomembranous colitis should be carried out.

Management

- Acute diarrhoea is self-limiting and requires no drug treatment.
- Dehydration should be treated with oral rehydration salts and plenty of fluids (first-line treatment).
- Drug treatment includes:
- antimotility drugs
- probiotics.

Antimotility drugs

- *Co-phenotrope* is a mixture of a synthetic opioid (diphenoxylate) and atropine. The atropine is present to avoid abuse of the drug.
- Prolonged usage of co-phenotrope can cause morphine-type dependence and therapy should be reviewed after 48 h.
- *Codeine phosphate* is also an opioid. The maximum dosage is 240 mg in 24 h.
- *Loperamide* is a synthetic opioid analogue but is relatively free from CNS opioid effects.
- It should be used with caution in liver disease as it is metabolised in the liver.
- The maximum dosage of loperamide is 16 mg in 24 h.

Probiotics

Probiotics are dietary supplements containing live bacteria or yeasts. They reflect the body's naturally occurring gut flora, such as the lactic acid bacteria.

- They have beneficial effects on health.
- Probiotics are of value in diarrhoea as they increase immune responses and will assist in re-establishing the natural gut flora.

Antibiotics

- Antimicrobial drugs are not recommended in gasteroenteritis.
- *Metronidazole* is the drug of choice in amoebic dysentery and *C. difficile* infection.
- Ciprofloxacin may be prescribed in patients presenting with dysentery or exposure to a bacterial infection. Before prescribing cipfrofloxacin, the following need to be taken into consideration:
- quinolones induce seizures in both epileptics and non-epileptics
- concurrent use of a NSAID may further enhance the tendency to seizures
- tendon damage can occur with quinolones
- ciprofloxacin is a cytochrome P-450 enzyme inhibitor and may interact with many other drugs.

> **Tip**
>
> Morphine can also be given for diarrhoea, but is not recommended as it causes significant constipation as a side-effect. It is susceptible to abuse and so requires monitoring.

Monitoring parameters

- Antimotility drugs should be avoided in children and in severe gastroenteritis or dysentery.
- Co-phenotrope should not be sold over the counter for use in patients under 16 years of age.
- Side-effects of co-phenotrope include the opioid side-effects such as constipation, nausea, vomiting, dry mouth and drowsiness.
- The side-effects of codeine phosphate include constipation, drowsiness, nausea and vomiting.
- Side-effects of loperamide include abdominal cramps, dizziness, drowsiness, urticaria.
- Alcohol must be avoided with metronidazole as the drug can cause a disulfiram type reaction.
- Ciprofloxacin may cause seizures and this is more likely if there is concurrent use of a NSAID.

Counselling

- Patients are advised to take plenty of fluids.
- Explaination of how to reconstitute oral rehydration salts should be given.
- Patients and family should be advised on hygiene and general handwashing.
- High-carbohydrate foods such as bread are recommended.

> **Tip**
>
> Diabetic patients should take care when using oral rehydration salt because of the glucose content; careful blood glucose monitoring should be emphasised.

Multiple choice questions

1. **Which of the following is *not* a side-effect of morphine?**
a. Drowsiness
b. Constipation
c. Taste disturbance
d. Dry mouth
e. Vomiting

2. **Are the following statements true or false?**
a. Probiotics have no benefit in diarrhoea.
b. The first-line treatment for diarrhoea is loperamide.
c. Dysentery is when there is blood with diarrhoea.
d. Antibiotics are used to treat dysentery.

Useful website

http://www.nhsdirect.nhs.uk

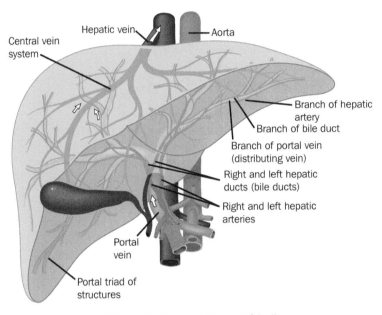

Figure 14.1 The internal anatomy of the liver.

Overview

- The liver is one of the largest organs of the body.
- Liver disease can be acute or chronic.
- Alcohol is the most common cause of liver disease in the Western world.
- Liver function tests are used in conjunction with imaging techniques to identify liver disease.
- Complications of liver disease include ascites, hepatic encephalopathy, portal hypertension and varices.

Aetiology

- The liver is one of the largest organs in the body and liver disease can be acute or chronic.
- Acute liver disease is self-limiting; in certain situations it may develop into acute liver failure.

- Chronic liver disease occurs over a long period of time and involves permanent changes to the structure of the liver and the hepatocytes.
- The liver has many functions, which can be affected to different degrees by liver disease:
- storage, e.g. glycogen
- secretion, e.g. bile salts
- synthesis, e.g. albumin
- metabolism, e.g. drugs
- clearance, e.g. aldosterone
- excretion, e.g. cholesterol
- homeostasis, e.g. glucose.
- Causes of liver disease include:
- viral infections: hepatitis A, B, C, D, E and G
- alcohol: most common cause of liver disease; approximately 25% of chronic alcoholics will develop liver disease
- immune disorders, e.g. autoimmune hepatitis
- genetic disorders, e.g. Wilson's disease
- Gilbert's syndrome.

Signs and symptoms

- Spider naevi
- Finger clubbing
- Gynaecomastia
- Loss of body hair
- Jaundice
- Enlarged liver
- Alopecia
- Palmar erythema
- White nails
- Ascities
- Portal hypertension
- Hepatic encephalopathy
- Pruritis.

Chronic complications of liver disease

Jaundice
Jaundice can be both an acute and a chronic sign of liver disease.
It occurs when serum bilirubin levels are high. Bilirubin is metabolised by the liver; therefore, it will accumulate if the liver is not functioning to its full capacity. It is clinically detectable when plasma bilirubin

is 35 μmol/L. Jaundice presents as yellowing of the skin, mucous membranes and iris.

Portal hypertension

Usual portal venous pressure is 2–5 mmHg. If this becomes chronically high, collateral veins can form. These can form throughout the body, but are found mainly in the GI tract. The presence of these veins allows portal blood to enter the systemic circulation directly, bypassing the liver. If the portal venous pressure remains high, this may lead to bleeding varices and is potentially life threatening. Portal hypertension also contributes to hepatic encephalopathy and ascites.

Ascites

Ascites is the accumulation of fluid in the abdominal cavity. In liver disease, there are three main causes of ascites:

- portal hypertension: altering capillary pressure and permeability, leading to the accumulation of fluid in the peritoneal cavity
- low blood albumin following reduced synthesis in the liver leads to fluid seepage from blood vessels
- aldosterone (the hormone responsible for fluid retention) accumulation when the damaged liver cannot metabolise it adequately.

Hepatic encephalopathy

Hepatic encephalopathy occurs in profound liver dysfunction. Neurotoxic substances enter directly into the brain, bypassing the damaged liver. Ammonia is one such substance and it alters the permeability of the blood–brain barrier. The patient presents with an altered mental state, euphoria and confusion. In severe cases, coma can be the end-result.

Gynaecomastia

The damaged liver is unable to metabolise oestrogen which can lead to feminisation in males. In women, it presents as irregular menstrual cycle and reduced fertility.

Investigations

Liver function tests

- Bilirubin is raised in hepatocellular damage, cholestasis and haemolysis.

Tips

Liver function tests alone cannot help diagnose the extent or the type of liver disease. They are a useful indicator to demonstrate poor liver function. Other tests such as imaging need to be used in conjunction to confirm diagnosis and classify the type of liver disease.

Liver function tests are of value once the patient is diagnosed and is being treated for liver disease. They should be monitored regularly to give an indication of disease progression and the effectiveness of drug and non-drug therapy.

- Transaminases: aspartate transaminase (AST) and alanine transaminase (ALT) are released from the liver in hepatocellular damage
- Alkaline phosphatase (ALP) is released in cholestasis.
- Albumin is synthesised in the liver. Serum albumin indicates the extent of chronic liver disease as it has a long half life (approx 20 days)
- Prothrombin time: clotting factors synthesised in the liver. Good indicator of acute liver damage due to short half life (about 6 h). In combination with albumin, gives a good indication of damage in both acute and chronic liver disease.

Liver biopsy

Liver biopsy is the gold standard in diagnosing the severity of chronic liver disease.

Management, monitoring and counselling

Ascities

- Sodium intake should be restricted to 60–90 mEq per day.
- Spironolactone (aldosterone antagonist) is the drug of choice. It can be used alone or with a loop diuretic.
- Side-effects of spironolactone include hyperkalaemia and gynaecomastia. The latter may be problematic as gynaecomastia is likely in patients with liver disease regardless of the use of spironolactone.
- Paracentesis can relieve abdominal pressure from ascites.
- Transjugular intrahepatic portosystemic stent shunt (TIPSS) is placed to provide portosystemic shunting to reduce portal pressure.
- Patients should be evaluated for liver transplant.
- Desired weight loss is 0.5–1 kg per day; water in versus water out should be monitored.

Portal hypertension

- Propranolol is the only beta-blocker licensed for portal hypertension. It is given to reduce portal venous pressure and prevent recurrent variceal bleeds.
- Adverse effects include vivid dreams, bradycardia, coldness of extremities, fatigue and bronchospasm.
- Patients should not stop taking this drug unless advised to do so by a doctor.

Hepatic encephalopathy

- Dietary protein intake should be reduced to 20 g per day.
- Lactulose, an osmotic laxative, reduces the pH of colonic content thus reducing colonic ammonia absorption; patients are monitored for two to three bowel motions a day.
- Metronidazole reduces ammonia production from GI bacteria.
- A disulfiram type reaction occurs if metronidazole is taken concurrently with alcohol.

Pruritis

- Pruritis can be a very distressing symptom of liver disease and requires reatment.
- Antihistamines are not very effective for pruritis in liver disease. If given, non-sedating antihistamines would be preferable (e.g. loratidine), as sedating antihistamines could mask the effects of hepatic encephalopathy.
- Anion exchange resins (colestyramine) bind to the bile acids that cause itching and is first-line therapy. Anion exchange resins can reduce the absorption of other drugs taken at the same time. Patients should be advised to take their drugs an hour before or 4 h after taking a dose of an anion exchange resin.
- Topical preparations such as calamine lotion can be used.

Oesophageal varices

- Vasopressin reduces portal blood flow and portal pressure; it is given IV to stop bleeding.
- Adverse effects of vasopressin include angina, myocardial infarction and arrhythmia.
- Vasopressin should not be used in patients with ischaemic heart disease. Glyceryl trinitrate can be given to overcome the cardiac side-effects.
- Terlipressin, given IV, is the drug of choice; it releases vasopression over several hours without the cardiac effects.
- Octreotide, given IV, stops variceal bleeding and reduces portal venous pressure.
- TIPSS is used for acute bleeding.
- Balloon tamponade is a short-term measure.
- Banding of varices together is the treatment of choice.

Clotting

- Treatment is vitamin K (pytomenadione), 10 mg given IV for 3 days.
- The patient's INR and prothrombin time are monitored.

Tips

NSAIDs and anticoagulants should be avoided in patients with liver disease, as they will have clotting abnormalities. NSAIDs may also cause variceal bleeding.

Sedative drugs such as opioids should also be avoided as they may precipitate and mask the signs of hepatic encephalopathy.

Multiple choice questions

1. **Which of the following is *not* a sign of liver disease?**
a. Spider naevi
b. Finger clubbing
c. Gynaecomastia
d. Taste disturbance
e. Itching

2. **Are the following statements true or false?**
a. Prothrombin has a long half life.
b. Terlipressin is the drug of choice for bleeding varices.
c. Alcohol is the most common cause of liver disease.
d. The liver stores water-soluble vitamins.

Useful website

http://www.nhsdirect.nhs.uk

The renal system

chapter 15
Acute renal failure

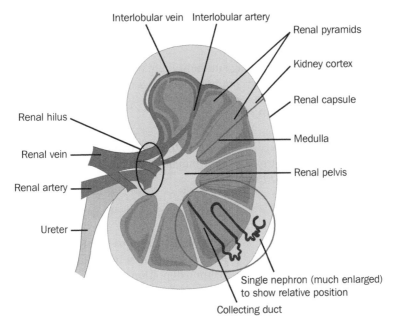

Figure 15.1 The kidney.

Interlobular vein Interlobular artery
Renal pyramids
Kidney cortex
Renal capsule
Renal hilus
Medulla
Renal vein
Renal pelvis
Renal artery
Ureter
Single nephron (much enlarged)
to show relative position
Collecting duct

Overview

- Acute renal failure occurs when the function of the kidneys declines rapidly.
- It can be classified into pre-renal, renal and post-renal types.
- Fluid electrolyte balance is affected.
- Treatment aims are to correct the fluid and electrolyte imbalances.

Aetiology

- Acute renal failure (ARF) is when the function of the kidneys declines rapidly over a period of days or weeks.
- Renal failure can be classified into three main types depending on whether the cause is before blood flow into the kidney, within the kidney or beyond the kidney in the urinary system.

- Pre-renal causes reduce renal perfusion, for example hypotension, hypovolaemia and drugs that reduce blood flow (e.g. ACE inhibitors).
- Intrinsic damage to the renal tissue occurs in diseases such as acute tubular necrosis (ATN), vascular disease and glomerulonephritis, or from nephrotoxic drugs (e.g. aminoglycosides).
- Post-renal causes include obstruction in the urinary tract (e.g. renal stones).
- ARF has an average mortality rate of 60%.
- ATN is the most common form of renal failure. It follows prolonged ischaemia as a result of pre-renal failure or direct damage. ATN causes include:
  - septic shock
  - nephrotoxic drugs (e.g. NSAIDs, ciclosporin, vancomicin, gentamicin, methotrexate), environmental toxins or microbial toxins
  - acute blood loss.

Signs and symptoms

Tip

Most patients are diagnosed in hospital through routine blood tests.

Signs and symptoms of ARF are non-specific. ARF can present with volume overload or volume depletion.
Signs and symptoms of ARF with volume depletion include:

- high serum creatinine
- high serum potassium
- high serum urea: uraemia causes nausea, muscle cramps, vomiting, decreased consciousness and GI bleeding
- increase in serum hydrogen ions (metabolic acidosis)
- increase in serum phosphate
- oliguria
- fluid loss
- thirst
- tachycardia
- hypotension.

Signs and symptoms of ARF with volume overload include:

- oedema
- weight gain
- dyspnoea (nocturnal)
- jugular venous distension.

Investigations

- Serum urea and creatinine are usually elevated.
- Urine output is reduced.

- Creatinine clearance (volume of serum that would be cleared of creatinine by excretion of urine over 1 min) can be calculated with the Cockcroft–Gault equation (Figure 15.2).

For males

$$\text{Creatinine clearance} = \frac{1.23 \times \text{Body weight} \times (140 - \text{age})}{\text{Serum creatinine}}$$

For females

$$\text{Creatinine clearance} = \frac{1.04 \times \text{Body weight} \times (140 - \text{age})}{\text{Serum creatinine}}$$

Figure 15.2 Calculation of creatinine clearance (mL/min) from serum creatinine (mmol/L) using the Cockcroft–Gault equation. The patient's age is expressed in years and body weight in kilograms.

Management

The aim of treatment is to prolong life, restore kidney function and prevent disease progression.

Correction of fluid and electrolyte balance

- Urea (increased, reduced excretion) is reduced by protein restriction.
- Potassium (increased, reduced excretion) can be reduced by dietary potassium restriction and stopping any potassium supplements or any drugs that can cause hyperkalaemia (spironolactone). Ion exchange resins (e.g. calcium resonium) will remove potassium slowly.
- Hydrogen ions (increased, reduced excretion, causing acidosis) can be 'mopped up' with sodium bicarbonate.
- Calcium (decreased, malabsorption) can be adjusted with oral calcium supplementation (rarely necessary).
- Phosphate (increased, reduced excretion) usually does not require treatment. If necessary, phosphate-binding agents such as Aludrox can be given.
- Fluids are given as sodium chloride 0.9%.
- If the kidneys do not respond to fluid therapy (lack of renal perfusion), loop diuretics, mannitol or dopamine can be tried to increase renal perfusion.

Dialysis

- Dialysis is indicated when life is at risk and renal function is poor enough to risk the patient's life.
- Dialysis removes toxins and excess fluids; it corrects fluid electrolyte imbalances and controls signs of sepsis.

Tips

Acidosis may precipitate hyperkalaemia. Hyperkalaemia can be life threatening as it can cause cardiac arrhythmias and may result in a cardiac arrest.

Treatment of life-threatening hyperkalaemia is with calcium gluconate 10% IV, which protects the heart, and insulin, which stimulates intracellular potassium uptake.

- There are four common types of dialysis:
  - haemodialysis
  - haemofiltration
  - haemodiafiltration
  - peritoneal dialysis.

Tip

Most drugs are cleared renally and some drugs are nephrotoxic. If a patient suffers with renal impairment, dosages need to be adjusted to avoid accumulation of the drug or further damage to the kidney. Some drugs may need to be avoided altogether (NSAIDs) as they may accelerate the patient into end-stage renal failure.

Monitoring parameters

- Urine output is monitored (fluid in versus fluid out).
- All electrolytes (e.g. potassium, hydrogen, phosphate, calcium) and urea and creatinine should be monitored regularly.
- The kidney is the main site for the excretion of drugs and toxins and dosages of other prescribed drugs should be adjusted accordingly.
- Nephrotoxic drugs should be avoided or doses significantly reduced.
- The kidney metabolises insulin and so dosage reductions will be needed.
- The kidney converts the inactive form of vitamin D to its active form (1,25-dihydroxycolecalciferol). Patients with ARF require vitamin D replacement therapy in the active form (alfacalcidol).

Multiple choice questions

1. Which of the following is *not* a sign or symptom of ARF with volume depletion?
a. Weight gain
b. Hyperkalaemia
c. Oliguria
d. Thirst
e. Tachycardia

2. Are the following statements true or false?
a. Potassium levels are high in ARF.
b. The patient may display signs of oliguria.
c. Insulin can be given to treat hyperkalaemia in an emergency.
d. Metabolic acidosis can occur.

Useful websites

http://www.pharmj.com
http://www.nhsdirect.nhs.uk

chapter 16

Chronic renal failure

Overview

- Chronic renal failure is long-term damage to the kidney and is irreversible.
- The presence of protein in the urine is a good indicator of chronic renal failure.
- Dialysis is considered for patients with very poor functioning kidneys.
- Anaemia, electrolyte disturbances and oedema are all signs of chronic renal failure.

Aetiology

- Chronic renal failure (CRF) is an irreversible progressive destruction of the kidneys.
- Protein may be present in the urine.
- CRF signifies the possibility of end-stage renal failure which can in turn give rise to cardiovascular disease.
- Damage occurs to the infrastructure of the kidney and nephrons are lost. The patient's glomerular filtration rate (GFR) can no longer be maintained and falls very quickly.
- Causes of CRF include:
- hypertension
- diabetes
- urinary obstruction
- nephrotoxic drugs.

Signs and symptoms

- Nausea and vomiting
- Anorexia
- Lethargy
- Peripheral neuropathy
- Pruritus
- Bruising
- Hypertension
- Anaemia: failure of erthyropoietin production
- Pericarditis
- Impotence
- Nocturia.

Tip

Electrolyte disturbances are the same in CRF as in acute renal failure (ARF) and the treatment regimen is identical. Sodium can be affected in CRF. The patient can have hypo- or hypernatraemia, or even normal serum sodium.

Investigations

- Structural assessment is by imaging procedures:
- ultrasonography
- intravenous urography
- radiography
- MRI or CT.
- Creatinine clearance is assessed using the Cockcroft–Gault equation (see Figure 15.2).

Management

- Aim of treatment is to relieve symptoms, stop the causative factor of CRF and prevent worsening of kidney function.
- Correction of electrolyte imbalance is the same as for ARF (Chapter 15).
- Dialysis is covered in Chapter 15.
- Renal transplant is the treatment for end-stage renal failure; patients will require long-term immunosupression (e.g. ciclosporin) after a transplant.

Tip

Haemodialysis and peritoneal dialysis may relieve many of the symptoms of CRF.

Management of symptoms

- Hypertension is covered in Chapter 2:
- diuretics (not potassium sparing) will be of benefit if oedema is present
- calcium-channel blockers
- alpha-blockers
- ACE inhibitors, but contraindicated in renal artery stenosis
- beta-blockers.
- Fluid restriction and sodium and potassium restriction are required.
- Pruritus can be relieved with antihistamines.
- Anaemia is treated with epoetin alpha and beta (human recombinant erythropoietins).
- Hyperparathyroidism is a consequence of increased calcium and active vitamin D; cinacalcet suppresses parathormone.

Monitoring parameters

- Urine output to be monitored (fluid in versus fluid out).
- All electrolytes (e.g. potassium, hydrogen, phosphate, calcium), urea and creatinine should be monitored regularly.
- Symptom monitoring should assess if they are getting better or worsening.
- Doses of other prescribed drugs should be adjusted accordingly.
- Nephrotoxic drugs should be avoided or doses significantly reduced.

- Sodium intake should be restricted to 80 mmol/day. Fluids should also be restricted; patient can suck on ice cubes to alleviate dry mouth symptoms.
- Diet should have restricted protein.
- Potassium-rich foods such as bananas, chocolate and beer should be avoided.
- The patient should understand the side-effects of any drugs prescribed (e.g. antihypertensive drugs or antihistamines).

Multiple choice questions

1. **Are the following statements true or false?**
a. A diet rich in protein should be given to patients with CRF.
b. NSAIDS should be avoided in patients with CRF.
c. Sodium levels can be high, low or remain normal.
d. ACE inhibitors can be given to patients with CRF providing the dose is reduced.

2. **Are the following statements regarding CRF true or false?**
a. Paracetamol is a nephrotoxic drug.
b. The Cockcroft–Gault equation gives an indication of serum creatinine levels.
c. Bruising may occur in patients with CRF.
d. Potassium levels are low in CRF.
e. The patient's GFR can be easily maintained.

Useful websites

http://www.pharmj.com
http://www.nhsdirect.nhs.uk

Infectious diseases

chapter 17

Tuberculosis

Overview

- Tuberculosis is an important cause of infection-related deaths worldwide.
- The incidence is increasing in the UK.
- It is treatable using a combination of antituberculosis agents.
- Treatment duration is greater than most other infections, at least 6 months.
- Adherence is very important to treatment outcome.
- Patients must be aware of the many potential adverse effects with antituberculosis agents.

Epidemiology

- Tuberculosis (TB) is the second leading cause of infection-related deaths worldwide, causing 1.7 million deaths in 2003.
- 30% of the world's population is thought to be infected with TB.
- The highest incidence is in sub-Saharan Africa, owing to the prevalence of HIV.
- In England and Wales, rates of TB declined steadily from 117 139 cases in 1913 to a low of 5086 cases in 1987. However, since then, numbers have risen annually, with 6837 cases being reported in 2003.
- Approximately 70% of cases in England and Wales occur in those born abroad.
- Other risk factors include HIV infection, immunosuppression, homelessness, chronic renal failure and alcohol and drug misuse.
- There are geographic variations within the UK, with London having the highest rate (41.3/100 000 population) and Northern Ireland having the lowest (3.3/100 000 population)
- Untreated TB has a poor prognosis, with 50% mortality rate within 2 years; however, most patients can be successfully treated with adequate chemotherapy.
- The incidence of drug resistance in TB is increasing worldwide. Multidrug-resistant strains of mycobacteria (MDR-TB) are responsible for approximately 10% of new cases in China and Eastern Europe and 1.3% of new cases in the UK.

Tip

TB is a notifiable disease. As such, all patients with a diagnosis of TB are reported to the local Consultant in Communicable Disease Control, who will investigate whether other individuals may be at risk and attempt to determine the source of the infection. Other notifiable diseases include rubella, mumps, measles, tetanus, meningitis and food poisoning.

Tip

Some medications can increase the risk of patients developing active TB, such as anti-tumour necrosis factor agents used in the treatment of inflammatory conditions. Therefore, these patients should be carefully monitored for signs of the disease prior to and throughout their therapy.

Aetiology

- TB is caused by bacteria of the *Mycobacterium tuberculosis* complex. The three that cause infection in humans are *M. tuberculosis*, *M. bovis* and *M. africanum*, with 98% of cases in the UK caused by *M. tuberculosis*.
- The main route of transmission is through inhalation of aerosolised droplets, measuring between 1 and 5 μm in diameter, from an infected person coughing, sneezing or talking.
- The incubation period from infection to clinically identifiable disease can range from 2 to 10 weeks.
- 30% of those exposed will become infected.
- Only 5–10% of those initially infected will develop an acute infection, with the remainder's host defences containing the infection, resulting in latent infection.
- Approximately 10% of those with latent infection will develop an active infection later in their lives.
- During the primary infection, the bacteria can be carried by macrophages to other parts of the body where they can cause infection or become latent.
- The most common site of disease is the lungs but over 40% of disease occurs at other sites.

Table 17.1 Sites of tuberculosis disease

Site of tuberculosis disease	No. cases	Percentage of total
Pulmonary	3907	59.4
Extrathoracic lymph nodes	1066	16.2
Pleural	484	7.4
Intrathoracic lymph nodes	475	7.2
Bone/joint	310	4.7
Gastrointestinal	227	3.5
Genitourinary	115	1.7
Miliary	106	1.6
Meninges	99	1.5
CNS	52	0.8
Other	513	7.8

Adapted from Department of Health. *Immunisation against Infectious Disease*.[1]

Signs and symptoms

Some signs and symptoms are specific to the site of infection; however, others are ubiquitous to the majority of cases.

General signs and symptoms:
- fatigue
- fever
- night sweats
- weight loss.

Pulmonary disease:
- persistent cough of greater than 2 weeks
- pleuritic chest pain
- shortness of breath
- haemoptysis
- 'chest infection' unresponsive to antibiotics.

CNS disease:
- headache
- neck stiffness
- seizures
- loss of consciousness
- motor or sensory defects.

Bone and joint disease:
- joint pain
- weakness and paralysis if spine involved.

Lymph gland disease:
- painless red lumps at lymph glands
- may indicate widespread disease.

Investigations

In individuals with clinical signs, a number of tests are performed to make a certain diagnosis.

Microbiological tests
- Microbiological tests are performed to assess whether a patient is infectious, determine whether their disease is caused by a TB-causing organism and assess to which drugs the organism is likely to be susceptible.
- Tests include microscopy, culture, drug sensitivity testing and strain typing.
- Sputum samples are usually taken from those with suspected respiratory disease, plus samples from other sites if thought to be site of disease (e.g. blood samples, cerebrospinal fluid (CSF), tissue samples).
- At least three samples are taken from relevant sites and assessed microscopically. Quickest and easiest methods include the use of Ziehl–Neelsen or fluorescent stains, which highlight the presence of acid-fast bacilli.
- Culture methods are normally required for extrapulmonary sites and may take between 1 and 6 weeks to yield a result.

- Polymerase chain reaction tests are also available, which can detect the presence of *M. tuberculosis* and the genes responsible for rifampicin resistance.
- Blood-based immunological tests have also been recently introduced: the T-spot TB and Quantiferon tests. These can differentiate between TB infection and previous BCG vaccination.

Tuberculin testing

- Tuberculin testing can be used to detect latent infection and previous vaccination. It is performed using a Mantoux test, where an intradermal injection of tuberculin purified protein derivative is given to the patient. This should produce a 7 mm bleb. The result is usually read 48 to 72 h after injection but can be done up to 96 h later.
- The size of the resulting induration indicates the patient's previous exposure to TB.
- 6 mm is negative and indicates the individual is unlikely to have been exposed to TB
- 6–15 mm indicates previous infection, vaccination or exposure to a non-tuberculosis mycobacterium
- 15 mm is suggestive of TB infection, and the patient should be investigated further.
- The test may be affected by glandular fever, viral infections, live viral vaccines in the previous 4 weeks, sarcoidosis, corticosteroids and immunosuppression.

Chest radiography

- The first change that can be seen is one (or more) ill-defined opacity, usually in the upper lung lobes.
- Other changes include pulmonary infiltration, cavitations, fibrosis, pleural effusion and pneumothorax.

Other investigations

- Full blood counts and renal and hepatic function should be assessed.
- Bone profile and inflammatory markers may be raised.
- In advanced disease, patients may have anaemia, low serum albumin and hypercalcaemia.
- Hyponatraemia may occur with CNS or adrenal disease.
- Miliary disease may cause pancytopenia and raised transaminases.

Management

Combination therapy using a number of active drugs is always used. This is to minimise the risk of resistance emerging during therapy and to reduce the course length. As TB can exist in a number of environments and with different rates of metabolic activity, a number of drugs are employed in its treatment.

- Treatment guidelines for the UK were published by the British Thoracic Society and updated by NICE.
- The recommended first-line regimen consists of rifampicin, isoniazid and pyrazinamide, with the addition of ethambutol if there is any suspicion of isoniazid resistance.
- Second-line drugs may be required in the presence of resistance, contraindication or intolerance to first-line agents. These include the aminoglycosides streptomycin and amikacin and the related drug capreomycin, the quinolones moxifloxacin and ofloxacin, the macrolides clarithromycin and azithromycin, cycloserine, protionamide, rifabutin, clofazimine and para-aminosalicylate
- When sensitive TB is treated fully, treatment consists of two phases: the initial phase of three or four drugs lasting for 2 months and the continuation phase consisting of rifampicin and isoniazid for 4 months.
- The total duration of therapy is usually 6 months for most forms of TB, but this may be extended in drug-resistant and meningeal TB to 12 or more months.
- Dosing is based on the patient's body weight, which may increase as a patient is successfully treated, requiring dose adjustment (Table 17.2).
- All first-line drugs are administered as single daily doses to aid compliance.
- Fixed dose combinations exist, containing two or three of the first-line drugs. Care must be taken when prescribing and supplying anti-TB medication to ensure that patients receive the correct medication at all stages of their therapy.

Tip

Anti-TB therapy is provided in specialist centres in the UK and is exempt from prescription charges.

- In renal impairment, dosage reductions may be required for isoniazid, ethambutol and pyrazinamide.
- In liver impairment, dosage reductions may be required for rifampicin and isoniazid.
- Corticosteroids may be used for their anti-inflammatory effects in the treatment of pericardial and meningeal TB. Higher doses are required in those patients receiving rifampicin as this increases steroid metabolism.

Table 17.2 Daily doses of first-line antituberculosis medication

Drug	Adult dose	Child dose
Rifampicin	450 mg if body weight < 50 kg 600 mg if > 50 kg	10 mg/kg
Isoniazid	300 mg	5–10 mg/kg
Pyrazinamide	1.5 g if body weight < 50 kg 2 g if > 50 kg	35 mg/kg
Ethambutol	15 mg/kg	15 mg/kg

- The first-line regimen is considered to be safe in patients who are pregnant or breast-feeding.
- In patients where compliance with daily dosing is thought to be poor, regimens consisting of intermittent thrice weekly dosing may be utilised.

Vaccination

Vaccination against TB is done through the use of a live, attenuated strain derived from *M. bovis*, the Bacillus Calmette–Guerin vaccine (BCG). It does not prevent TB infection but provides some protection against the serious disseminated forms of the disease, such as miliary TB and meningitis. In the UK, the recommendations for BCG vaccination have recently changed and now target those at the highest risk of developing severe disease or being exposed for the first time, including:

- all infants 12 months old living in areas of the UK with an annual TB incidence 40 cases/100 000 population
- all infants and those under 5 years not previously vaccinated with a parent or grandparent from a country with an incidence of 40 cases/100 000 population
- those at occupational risk, such as healthcare workers with patient contact.

Monitoring

The efficacy of therapy is assessed through the use of sputum examination and culture. Patients with sensitive disease should become culture negative within 2 weeks of treatment. Monitoring of inflammatory markers, such as ESR, may also prove useful in measuring response to therapy.

Anti-TB therapy is associated with many adverse effects (Table 17.3). Patients should be monitored regularly for the presence of these and up to

Table 17.3 Main adverse effects of antituberculosis agents

Drug	Adverse effect
Rifampicin	Hepatitis, rash, GI disturbance, febrile illnesses
Isoniazid	Hepatitis, rash, peripheral neuropathy
Pyrazinamide	Nausea, anorexia, flushing, hepatitis, arthralgia, hyperuricaemia, gout, rash
Ethambutol	Ocular toxicity, arthralgia
Aminoglycosides	Tinnitus, ataxia, renal impairment
Protionamide	GI disturbance, hepatitis
Quinolones	Headache, drowsiness, fits
Macrolides	GI disturbances
Clofazimine	Headache, GI disturbance, red skin discoloration
Para-aminosalicylate	GI disturbance, hepatitis, rash
Cycloserine	Depression, fits, thyroid dysfunction

10% of patients on first-line treatment are thought to experience significant adverse effects.

- Drug-induced hepatitis is a potentially serious adverse effect and can be important to the outcome of therapy. Patients should be aware that any early signs of hepatitis such as nausea, anorexia and yellowing of the eyes must be reported.
- Baseline and regular assessment of liver function tests is also useful in monitoring patients for hepatitis. Transient mild elevations in liver function tests are to be expected and require further monitoring, but significant elevations in transaminases (5 times upper limit of normal (ULN)) require discontinuation of hepatitis-inducing agents.
- If drug-induced hepatitis occurs, therapy is usually withdrawn and gradually introduced agent by agent once the hepatitis has subsided. The offending drug can often be identified and omitted. These patients may require the use of additional anti-TB drugs and extended treatment durations. Single drugs should never be used alone.
- The relatively common side-effect of peripheral neuropathy with isoniazid is caused by depletion of vitamin B_6 and can be minimised through pyridoxine supplementation.
- Patients should have their vision checked prior to therapy with ethambutol and be told to report any changes in their vision. As treatment with ethambutol is normally only for the 2 months of the initial treatment phase, routine monitoring in not normally necessary.
- Drug interactions are common and often clinically significant with rifampicin and isoniazid.
- Rifampicin is a potent inducer of CYP450 isoenzymes and may cause decreases in the plasma levels of drugs such as antiretroviral drugs, antifungal agents, hormone therapies, including the contraceptive pill and levothyroxine, anticoagulants, anticonvulsants, corticosteroids and digoxin.
- Isoniazid is a relatively potent inhibitor of CYP450 isoenzymes and may interact with drugs such as phenytoin, carbamazepine, valproate, warfarin and theophylline.

Counselling

- Patients undergoing anti-TB therapy require extensive and comprehensive counselling prior to and throughout their treatment.
- Adherence is a major concern as inadequate therapy can result in treatment failure, increased period of infectiousness and the emergence of resistant strains.

Tip

It is important to provide anti-TB medication in the most appropriate form for the patient. This may require the use of extemporaneous manufactured liquids and unlicensed injections.

- Patient may fail to adhere for reasons such as the number of medications they are required to take, discontinuation when they feel better, the presence of adverse effects or poor understanding of their treatment.
- Strategies to improve compliance must focus on all these factors. Providing written education and information is useful.
- Patients should be educated to the main points of their treatment and the individual drugs they are taking.
- They should be told to report any adverse effects to their medical team as soon as it becomes apparent.

Multiple choice questions

1. Which of the following is *not* a symptom of TB?
a. Fever
b. Chronic cough
c. Weight gain
d. Night sweats
e. Haemoptysis

2. Are the following statements true or false?
a. Ethambutol may cause drug-induced hepatitis.
b. BCG vaccination does not prevent the pulmonary form of the disease.
c. Treatment duration is at least 6 months.
d. Rifampicin increases the effect of warfarin.
e. First-line anti-TB drugs may be used in pregnancy.

Reference

1. Department of Health (2006). *Immunisation against Infectious Disease*. London: Department of Health.

Useful websites

www.brit-thoracic.org.uk
www.nice.org
www.dh.gov.uk/greenbook

chapter 18

Bacterial infections

Overview

- Bacterial infections can cause significant morbidity and mortality.
- Commensal bacteria are present at many sites of the body.
- Infections often occur when the body's natural defences are impaired, for example when immunosuppressed or after surgery.
- Ideally, the narrowest spectrum and safest antibiotic should be used for the shortest duration.
- Empirical therapy is often undertaken when the causative organism is not known and relies on knowledge of likely causative organisms and spectrum of activity of antibiotics.
- Inappropriate usage of antibiotics has helped to contribute to increasing resistance amongst pathogenic bacteria.

Aetiology

- Many species of bacteria are carried naturally by the body.
- The majority do not cause disease under normal circumstances.
- Many bacteria are beneficial to bodily functions and are considered commensal flora. They assist in digestion and help to prevent infection from pathogenic bacteria.
- Some bacteria can be commensal bacteria in one part of the body but cause infection in other parts of the body; for example *Escherichia coli* is an intestinal commensal but a significant cause of urinary-tract infections and *Staphylococcus aureus* may be a skin commensal but cause wound infections.
- There are many types of bacterial infection. Any part of the body can become infected by the invasion of pathogenic bacteria when circumstances permit.
- For infection to occur, pathogenic bacteria must first become established at the site of infection and avoid the body's barriers to infection. This includes the immune system, physical barriers such as the skin, mucous membranes and commensal bacteria.
- The organisms that cause infection vary with the site of infection. Each type of infection is associated with a number of species; examples are given in Table 18.1.

Table 18.1 Common infections and the commonest causative organism

Site of infection	Infection	Common causative organisms
GI tract	Antibiotic-associated colitis	Clostridium difficile
	Bacterial gastroenteritis	Escherichia coli, Campylobacter jejuni, Shigella spp., Salmonella spp.
	Peptic ulcer	Helicobacter pylori
Cardiovascular system	Endocarditis	Enterococcus faecalis, Enterococcus faecium, Staphylococcus aureus, viridans streptococci
Respiratory tract	Community-acquired pneumonia	Streptococcus pneumoniae, Haemophilus influenzae, Moraxella catarrhalis, Mycoplasma pneumoniae
Urinary tract	Urinary-tract infection	Escherichia coli, Klebsiella spp.
Central nervous system	Meningitis	Streptococcus pneumoniae, Neisseria meningitidis, Haemophilus influenzae
Skin and soft tissue	Cellulitis	Staphylococcus aureus, Streptococcus pyogenes

Epidemiology

- It is difficult to determine the incidence of many common infections.
- Data are only collected routinely for certain serious infections such as meticillin-resistant *S. aureus* (MRSA) and *Clostridium difficile* in hospitalised patients and bacterial meningitis.
- Urinary-tract infections are one of the commonest bacterial infections in the UK, with half of all women receiving treatment at least once in their lives.
- There are approximately 2000 cases of bacterial meningitis in the UK each year.
- General risk factors for bacterial infections include:
- immunosuppression from disease or medication
- reduced immunity in the young and elderly
- malnutrition
- surgery
- prosthetic devices, such as hip replacements or heart valves
- diabetes mellitus
- burns.
- There are specific risk factors for each type of infection, such as lower respiratory tract infection in chronic obstructive pulmonary disease and urinary-tract infections with urinary catheter use.

Signs and symptoms

Some signs and symptoms are common to the majority of bacteria infections. These include:

- fever
- tachycardia
- sweating
- hypotension
- nausea and vomiting.

Specific infections may have typical signs or symptoms:

- local pain, inflammation and purulent discharge in soft tissue or ocular infections
- pain on micturition with a urinary-tract infection
- purulent or increased sputum in respiratory tract infection
- diarrhoea with GI infections
- seizures and photophobia in meningitis.

Investigations

- The investigations undertaken will depend upon the likely source of infection and the severity of the infection.
- In some infections it is possible to make a diagnosis and initiate treatment based on signs and symptoms and it is unnecessary to undertake further investigations, such as superficial, localised infections like conjunctivitis.
- For most other infections, a number of investigations will be undertaken with the aims of determining the source of the infection, the causative organism and the severity of the infection.
- The tests used depend on the infection but include:
- 'vital signs': temperature, pulse, blood pressure, respiratory rate
- white blood cell count would usually show an elevation, but chronic infection may result in decreased neutrophils
- inflammatory markers. CRP and ESR are usually raised.
- Samples from the likely site of infection may be taken for microbiological analysis (e.g. blood, CSF or urine samples). Tests on these include microscopic visualisation, often after staining, attempts to grow a culture of the organism and testing for antibiotic sensitivity.
- Radiographic imaging such as with X-ray or MRI can determine the extent or location of infection.
- Renal and hepatic impairment will require dosage adjustment for many antibiotics. Renal and hepatic impairment may also be caused by systemic bacterial infection.

Tips

Examples of common infections and their usual empiric treatments, including options in those with penicillin allergy, can be found in Chapter 5 of the BNF.

Many patients report that they are allergic to penicillins. However, many patients have actually only suffered mild intolerances, such as diarrhoea or nausea with previous courses. An assessment of the presence and type of previous reactions should always be undertaken prior to making decisions on antibiotic therapy.

Management

The goals of treatment are to:

- eradicate the causative organism
- prevent complications of infection
- minimise adverse effects from therapy.

The selection of antibiotic therapy is complex and depends upon the specific infection but some principles are common in all bacterial infections.

- If possible, an antibiotic should be selected that is known to be active against the causative organism. Usually this is not possible as the causative organism or its antibiotic sensitivity is not known. Consequently, an antibiotic is selected that is active against the likely pathogen; this is termed empirical therapy (Table 18.2).
- Patient-specific factors should be considered. These include comorbidities, concurrent medications, previous intolerances, renal and liver function, age and sex.
- The severity of the infection will contribute to selection of antibiotic therapy. In serious infections, it may be appropriate to start with potentially more toxic but more effective antibiotics until the causative organism is known.
- The route of treatment is determined by the availability of antibiotics to treat the infection and the severity of the infection. In severe infections, such as meningitis, it is common to initiate therapy via the IV route to achieve rapid and predictable systemic antibiotic levels.
- The dose of chosen antibiotic to be used depends on factors such as the patient's age, weight, renal and liver function, the severity and site of infection and the route of administration. The dose should be appropriate to treat the infection while minimising adverse effects to the patient.
- The duration of therapy is determined by the nature of the infection and the response to treatment. Some infections may require a

Table 18.2 Common infections and usual empiric therapy

Infection	Common antibiotic choices
Antibiotic-associated colitis	Metronidazole
Bacterial gastroenteritis	Usually self-limiting but erythromycin or ciprofloxacin may be used
Peptic ulcer	Combination of a proton pump inhibitor with two of amoxicillin, metronidazole and clarithromycin
Endocarditis	Dependent upon organism, includes benzylpenicillin, flucloxacillin or vancomycin; often with gentamicin
Community acquired pneumonia	Amoxicillin ± clarithromycin
Urinary tract infection	Trimethoprim or nitrofurantoin
Meningitis	Cefotaxime
Cellulitis	Flucloxacillin

single dose, such as urinary-tract infection, whereas others may require months of therapy, such as osteomyelitis.

- Some infections may be treated with one antibiotic but combination therapy is required in others. Comedication may be used in an attempt to reduce infection, to benefit from synergistic activity or because more than one antibiotic is required to cover all the causative organisms.

Monitoring parameters

- The efficacy of antibiotic therapy is assessed using the same tests as for identifying the presence and severity of infection. Again the types of measurement used depend upon the location and severity of infection.
- Superficial infections such as conjunctivitis require only a check on the resolution of symptoms, whereas severe systemic infections, such as meningitis, require more intensive monitoring.
- The improvement in visual indicators is a simple method of assessment, such as decrease in erythema in cellulitis or purulence in soft tissue infections.
- Measurement of vital signs can be used to monitor progress.
- Laboratory tests, such as white cell count and inflammatory markers, are used to monitor response to treatment.
- Improvements in symptoms can be used to determine improvement, for example decrease in breathlessness in pneumonia or decrease in local pain on passing urine in urinary-tract infections.
- Specific monitoring may be required for the antibiotics that are being used.
- Penicillin-type antibiotics can be associated with allergic reactions, even in those having previously received them safely. Patients should be monitored for signs such as rash, breathlessness and wheeze.
- Some antibiotics require monitoring of their plasma levels to determine the most appropriate dose for the patient, to ensure a high enough level for efficacy without reaching potentially toxic doses.
- Knowledge of potential adverse effects is required for each antibiotic used, to ensure that drug-specific monitoring is

Tip

There are few treatments for infections that can be provided without prescription. Trimethoprim is commonly used in the treatment of simple, self-limiting urinary-tract infections in females. It is currently proposed that it should be available for this indication as an over-the-counter preparation. If this occurs, it will become the first systemic antibiotic to be available in such a way in the UK.

Tip

Some antibiotics have a narrow therapeutic window but are used in clinical practice when the benefits outweigh the risks. Examples include the glycopeptide vancomycin and the aminoglycosides such as gentamicin. These are often required for the treatment of otherwise resistant infections. Vancomycin is the first-line treatment for systemic MRSA infections but is associated with renal and ototoxicity. For this reason, plasma levels must be closely monitored during treatment.

undertaken, such as monitoring of liver function tests with rifampicin.

Counselling

- Patients should be provided with specific information relating to their infection and its management.
  - In general, they should be aware of how to take their specific antibiotic therapy and its likely adverse effects (e.g. the need to avoid alcohol with metronidazole).
  - They should be told to complete the recommended course, irrespective of whether they feel better.
  - They should take their antibiotics at regular intervals, for example twice daily should be as close to 12 hourly as possible.
  - They should be told how to take their antibiotics for the best effect, for example with meals or on an empty stomach.
- They should be made aware of potential drug interactions, especially broad-spectrum antibiotics and the contraceptive pill.
- It may take a number of days before the effects of antibiotics become apparent.
- Reinforcement that antibiotics are not effective for the treatment of viral infections, such as the common cold, should be given when appropriate.
- Patients should be aware of the need to seek medical attention in the event of serious adverse effects, such as severe rash or breathlessness.

> **Tip**
>
> Antibiotic resistance is a significant public health issue. Measures employed to reduce resistance include the avoidance of antibiotics for viral and self-limiting infections, using the shortest course possible and placing limits on their use in animals.

Multiple choice questions

1. **Which of the following is *not* a risk factor for bacterial infection?**
a. Immunosuppression in disease or medication
b. Obesity
c. Surgery
d. Diabetes mellitus
e. Burns

2. **Are the following statements true or false?**
a. Vancomycin requires monitoring of plasma levels to reduce the risk of hepatotoxicy.
b. Alcohol should be avoided when taking metronidazole.
c. *E. coli* commonly causes urinary-tract infections but is naturally present in the GI tract.

d. Empiric therapy is using antibiotics that are active against the most likely pathogens when the exact causative organism is unknown.

e. Patients diagnosed with bacterial gastroenteritis should receive prompt antibiotic therapy.

Useful websites

www.nice.org.uk
www.bsac.org.uk

The central nervous system

chapter 19

Epilepsy

Overview

- Epilepsy is the tendency to have seizures, which are triggered by abnormal electrical discharges in the brain.
- There are two main types of seizures: generalised and partial.
- Treatment is based on the type of seizure, which is diagnosed using MRI and electroencephalography.
- Treatment aims include preventing a seizure and suppressing the abnormal discharges in the brain.
- Healthcare professionals are required to help the patient to understand the disease and the medication they are taking; monitoring is required as treatment is long term (at least 3 years).

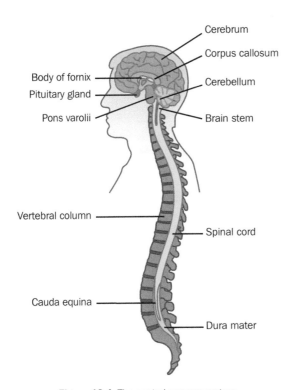

Figure 19.1 The central nervous system.

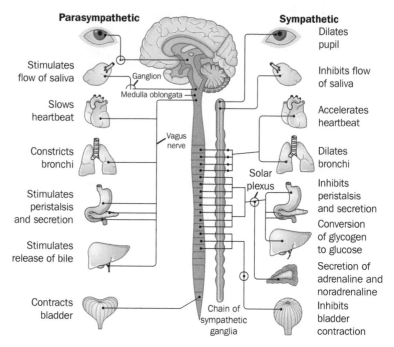

Parasympathetic

Sympathetic

Dilates
pupil

Stimulates
flow of saliva

Ganglion

Inhibits flow
of saliva

Medulla oblongata

Slows
heartbeat

Accelerates
heartbeat

Vagus
nerve

Constricts
bronchi

Dilates
bronchi

Solar
plexus

Inhibits
peristalsis
and secretion

Stimulates
peristalsis
and secretion

Conversion
of glycogen
to glucose

Stimulates
release of bile

Secretion of
adrenaline and
noradrenaline

Contracts
bladder

Chain of
sympathetic
ganglia

Inhibits
bladder
contraction

Figure 19.2 Function of the central nervous system.

Tips

A single seizure does not indicate epilepsy; further investigations should be carried out as to the cause of the seizure as many conditions have seizures as a symptom.

Recurrent seizures would be typical in patients with epilepsy.

Aetiology

- Epilepsy is a tendency to have seizures.
- Seizures are triggered by abnormal electrical discharges in the brain.
- Epileptic seizures present as various types depending on the origin of the electrical discharge: whether it is localised or widespread.
- Causes vary widely: head injury, alcohol abuse, brain tumours, infection, cerebrovascular disease and genetic factors.
- Epilepsy from trauma at birth can still initiate in adulthood.

Epidemiology

- Epileptic seizures are common.
- The risk of having epilepsy at some point in life is between 2% and 5%.
- Up to 5% of the population will have at least one seizure in their lifetime.

- Approximately 75% of people with epilepsy will become seizure free at some point in their life but 25% of patients will suffer with chronic epilepsy.
- There is increased mortality in patients with epilepsy; common causes of death include status epilepticus, head injury, tumours and road traffic accidents. Sudden unexplained death is common, especially in chronic epilepsy.

Signs and symptoms

- Signs and symptoms of epilepsy depend on the type of epilepsy.
- There are two main types of seizure: generalised and partial.
- Within these types are a number of subtypes (Table 19.1).

Table 19.1 Seizures

Type of seizure	Symptoms	Any other information
Generalised	Impaired consciousness from onset	The electrical abnormal discharge involves both hemispheres of the brain
Tonic–clonic (grand mal)	Fall, stiffness, pupil dilates, frothing at the mouth, jerking muscles, biting the tongue, pallor and whole body spasms	Symptoms occur without any prior warning; symptoms last a few minutes after which the patient may feel confused and go into a deep sleep
Absence (petit mal)	Blank stare, rolling of eyes and moving lips	Common in childhood; lasts only a few seconds; child may not recall having the seizure
Myoclonic	Rapid muscular contractions, jerks in facial and pelvic muscles	Usually occurs in the morning; immediate recovery
Atonic	Sudden loss of muscle tone, falling to the ground	Quick recovery; rare type of seizure
Partial		Abnormal discharge originating from a focal part of the brain
Simple partial	Conscious, stiffness of one part of the body, jerking	Usually progresses to other partial seizures
Complex partial	Smacking of lips, repetitive behaviour (e.g. walking in a circle), visual hallucinations, semiconscious	May progress to secondary generalised seizures
Secondary generalised	May have an aura; symptoms are the same as a generalised tonic–clonic seizure	Abnormal discharge originates at a focal point in the brain and then spreads to the entire brain

Diagnosis

Diagnosis should be made by a specialist.
The following should be documented before confirming a diagnosis:
- detailed history and symptoms of the attack by the patient

■ detailed history of the seizure/convulsion by an eye witness (usually a relative)

■ for some complex cases, recording the patient can be of use.

Investigations

■ Electroencephalography (EEG) records abnormal neuronal discharge and helps determine seizure type.

■ MRI is the investigation of choice, especially when structural abnormalities are suspected.

■ CT is used if MRI is contraindicated or in acute cases.

Tips

An EEG should not be used alone to confirm the diagnosis of epilepsy.
Once an MRI or EEG is ordered, the test should be performed within 4 weeks (UK government initiative).

Management

■ Aim of treatment is to suppress abnormal electrical discharges and prevent the epileptic seizures.

■ Therapy is long term, a minimum of 3–4 years.

■ The aim is to control seizures with one drug with the fewest side-effects possible; monotherapy is preferred.

■ If monotherapy with a particular drug fails, monotherapy with another antiepileptic drug should be considered.

■ Treatment should be initiated slowly, titrating the dose gradually; rapid introduction of the drugs may induce side-effects.

■ Choice of treatment depends on the type of seizure, other comorbidities, other drug treatment, patient choice and lifestyle.

■ Patient needs to be monitored closely while on maintenance treatment.

■ Therapy can be withdrawn, after discussion with patient and carers, if the patient has been seizure free for 2 years or more. Therapy needs to be withdrawn slowly over 2–3 months.

Monitoring parameters

Side-effects of specific drugs used in epilepsy are given in Table 19.2.

Tip

Drug interactions are very common with antiepileptic drugs. Some induce the metabolism of other drugs; some may be susceptible to inhibition themselves. Appendix 1 of the BNF gives a list of such drug interactions.

Counselling

■ The condition and how to deal with it should be explained to the patient and/or the carer, including the type of seizures.

Table 19.2 Antiepileptic drugs

Antiepileptic drug	Indication	Side-effects	Other information
Acetazolamide	Adjuvant for tonic–clonic and partial seizures	Double vision, somnolence, rash, dizziness, loss of appetite, depression, headache, irritability	
Carbamazepine[a]	Generalised tonic–clonic and partial seizures	Urticaria, blurred vision, double vision, nausea	Used as monotherapy TDM indicated; monitor every 6–12 months once stabilised. Exhibits autoinduction
Clobazam	Used as an adjuvant	Drowsiness	May develop tolerance to this effect as treatment continues
Clonazepam	Used in all form of epilepsies and seizures	Fatigue, somnolence	Transient side-effects that disappear as treatment continues/dose reduces
Ethosuximide	Absence seizures	Headache, nausea, weight loss	Used as monotherapy; may be an adjuvant in other forms of seizures which occur with absence seizures
Gabapentin	Adjuvant in partial seizures, with or without secondary generalisation	Fatigue, headache, somnolence	
Lamotrigine	Monotherapy of partial seizures, primary and secondary tonic–clonic	Double vision, rash, headache, tiredness, hallucinations	Skin rash appears within 8 weeks of starting treatment but reverses on drug withdrawal. May be used as an adjuvant
Levetiracetam	Add-on therapy in the treatment of partial-onset seizures with or without secondary generalised tonic–clonic seizures	Somnolence, confusion, ataxia, tremor, irritability, headache	
Oxcarbazepine[a]	Partial seizures with or without secondary generalised tonic–clonic seizures	Headache, nausea, double vision, ataxia, confusion	Monotherapy or adjunctive therapy in adults and in children over 6 years
Phenobarbital[a]	All forms of epilepsy except absence seizures	Mental depression, drowsiness	

Table 19.2 (continued)

Phenytoin[a]	Tonic–clonic and or partial seizures	Gum hyperplasia, hirsutism, nystagmus, rash, blood dyscrasias, ataxia	TDM indicated; monitor every 6–12 months once stabilised
Primidone[a]	Generalised tonic–clonic	Drowsiness, listlessness	
Sodium valproate	Generalised and partial epilepsy	Weight gain, hair loss, irregular periods, blood dyscrasias	Hair regrowth occurs after 6 months. Patients should report any signs of infection/sore throat. Any problems with menstrual cycle should be reported to GP. TDM indicated if suspected toxicity
Tiagabine	Add-on therapy for partial seizures with or without secondary generalisation	Tiredness, dizziness, nervousness, low mood, difficulty concentrating	
Topiramate[a]	Partial seizures with or without secondary generalised seizures; seizures associated with Lennox–Gastaut syndrome; primary generalised tonic–clonic seizures	Somnolence, weight loss, dizziness, headache, paraesthesia	
Vigabatrin	Monotherapy in the treatment of infantile spasms; add-on therapy for resistant partial epilepsy with or without generalisation	Somnolence, depression, nausea, agitation, visual field defects	Visual field tests to be carried out every 6 months
Zonisamide	Adjuvant therapy in all partial seizures	Somnolence, headache, depression, nausea, agitation	

TDM, therapeutic drug monitoring.
[a]Cytochrome P-450 enzyme inducer.

- Drug treatment should be explained including the indications and the side-effects.
- If therapeutic drug monitoring is required, patients and carers should be advised on when to come for blood tests.
- Any likely drug interactions should be explained.
- The patient and carer should be directed to resources on epilepsy and given a named contact on the healthcare team for any further questions or problems that they wish to discuss.
- Any known triggers and how to avoid them should be explained.
- Safety in the home and any first-aid techniques should be outlined.
- Follow-up appointments are important to assess the patient's condition. The importance of adhering to these appointments must be stressed.
- Patients should adhere to their therapy. Formulations should not be changed unless advised by the doctor or pharmacist, as the dosage would need to be changed because of differences in bioavailability.

Multiple choice questions

1. Which of the following is *not* used for the treatment of generalised tonic-clonic seizures?
a. Phenytoin
b. Ethosuximide
c. Sodium valproate
d. Clobazam
e. Lamotrigine

2. Are the following statements true or false?
a. Phenytoin is an enzyme P-450 inhibitor.
b. Up to 15% of people suffer with a seizure in their lifetime.
c. Tonic-clonic seizures are also known as 'grand mal' seizures.
d. EEGs are used to diagnose epilepsy.

Useful websites

http://www.nice.org.uk
http://www.nhsdirect.nhs.uk
http://www.epilepsy.org.uk/
http://www.epilepsyresearch.org.uk

Overview

- Parkinson's disease is a progressive neurodegenerative disorder resulting mainly from the loss of dopamine in the substantia nigra.
- There is no cure or therapy able to halt its progression.
- Therapy is targeted at managing the symptoms, the main ones being tremor, rigidity and bradykinesia.
- Initial therapy aims to increase the amount of available dopamine.

Aetiology

- In Parkinson's disease, there is a deficiency in the neurotransmitter dopamine as a consequence of degenerative of dopaminergic neurones.
- A loss of approximately 80% of dopaminergic neurones is required before symptoms are observed.
- The damage occurs in nigrostriatial pathway, which ascends from the substantia nigra to the corpus striatum.
- The dopaminergic pathway usually has an inhibitory effect on the extrapyramidal motor system.
- Acetylcholine is the main excitatory neurotransmitter in this pathway and its effects are exaggerated as available dopamine reduces.
- There is also a loss of other neurones in the brain, including GABAergic, noradrenergic and serotonergic neurones, which helps to explain the presence of other symptoms and the lack of efficacy of dopamine replacement of these other symptoms.
- Pathologically, there are Lewy bodies in the substantia nigra.

Epidemiology

- Approximately 120 000 people in the UK are diagnosed with Parkinson's disease.
- It is slightly more common in men than women, at a ratio of 1.2:1.
- The prevalence increases with age, overall prevalence is 1 in 500 in the general adult population, 1 in 300 in those in their 60s and increasing to 1 in 80 in those over 80 years of age.

Tip

Many drugs can induce Parkinson-like symptoms. These include phenothiazines, metoclopramide, calcium-channel blockers, lithium, pethidine, amiodarone, valproate and selective serotonin-reuptake inhibitors (SSRIs). Patients should be aware of this prior to starting these drugs and told to seek medical advice if the adverse effect occurs. It is more common in the elderly and in females.

- There are approximately 10 000 newly diagnosed patients in the UK each year.
- The causes of Parkinson's disease are not yet fully understood but both environmental and genetic causes have been implicated.
- First-degree relatives have twice the risk of developing the condition.
- Pollutants, toxins, pesticides and smoking have been linked with an increased incidence.

Signs and symptoms

There are significant differences in the manner of presentation of Parkinson's disease in different patients; however, the three key symptoms occur:
- bradykinesia
- rigidity
- tremor.

Bradykinesia

- The main presentation involves bradykinesia, a slowing of movements, with associated hypokinesia, a reduction in movement.
- These can result in feelings of physical tiredness; because of the very gradual onset of the symptoms, it may be some time before a patient recognises that there may be an underlying problem rather than just the slowing down associated with getting older.
- In addition to affecting the limbs, hypokinesia can also affect the facial muscles leading to a bland expression that impairs communication.
- Fine movements may become more difficult; fatigue may occur and there may be a reduction in the amplitude of movement.

Rigidity

- Many patients are less aware of rigidity as it is difficult for them to distinguish as a separate symptom from their bradykinesia.
- Rigidity is present as a muscle resistance during passive movement, such as occurs when a third party moves one of the patient's limbs.
- It may result in external signs of Parkinson's disease such as a twisted neck or bent wrist.

Tremor

- Tremor is a classic, though not ubiquitous, symptom of Parkinson's disease, which is present in approximately three quarters of patients.
- Tremor is usually relatively coarse and is most prominent at rest.
- It can affect any muscles but commonly affects the thumb and forefinger, termed 'pill-rolling'.
- Tremor is often the symptom that causes the patient to refer themselves for medical review, leading to diagnosis.
- There are many other symptoms that may be associated with Parkinson's disease, including:
  - 'cogwheeling' may occur when significant tremor and rigidity are present
  - micrographia, where a patient's writing becomes much smaller and shakier than usual
  - postural instability owing to the inability to make fast subtle changes in reflexes, hence an increased risk of falls
  - gait changes such as shuffling while walking and a stooped posture
  - movement freezing prior to its normal completion
  - depression, common in those with Parkinson's disease.
- Less-common symptoms, often occurring with more advanced disease, include dysphagia, hallucinations, dementia, constipation, bladder problems, speech problems, sleep disturbance and sexual problems.

Investigations

- Making a definite diagnosis of Parkinson's disease is very difficult as there is no accurate clinical diagnostic test.
- The only accurate test is to determine the presence of Lewy bodies in the substantia nigra at autopsy.
- Diagnosis is usually made on the presence of signs and symptoms, with a lack of any other cause of these symptoms.
- Diagnostic tools can be used, such as the UK Parkinson's Disease Society Brain Bank Criteria. This features a number of inclusion, exclusion and supportive criteria to make a diagnosis.
- A trial of levodopa or apomorphine has been used to determine whether patients with suspected Parkinson's disease show a response, but this is not recommended.

Tip

The diagnosis of Parkinson's disease is very difficult to achieve conclusively. At autopsy, it is found that approximately 10–25% of those who had been diagnosed as having Parkinson's disease had been misdiagnosed.

- Patients diagnosed with Parkinson's disease should have their diagnosis reviewed regularly, especially if any atypical symptoms present.
- Imaging may be used to distinguish between Parkinson's disease and some similarly presenting conditions. A number of imaging techniques may be utilised, including CT and MRI and the visualisation of dopamine transporters using radioisotope-labelled dopamine-transporter ligands.

Tips

'Drug holidays' where patients have their therapy withdrawn for a period of time and then reintroduced is not recommended in routine practice because of the risk of neuroleptic malignant syndrome. This is a life-threatening condition characterised by muscle rigidity, fever, autonomic instability, cognitive instability and raised creatine kinase.

Problems often occur when patients are admitted to hospital or care homes. It is important that patients receive their antiparkinsonian medication at the correct times, and that they are only adjusted after consultation with a specialist in Parkinson's disease.

Management

- The aim of treatment is currently to control symptoms and minimise adverse effects from therapy.
- At present, there are no treatments that prevent the degeneration of the neurones or replace damaged neurones.
- No one treatment is appropriate as the initial therapy for all patients.
- The decision on which agent to use as initial therapy must be made after careful assessment of the patient, including which symptoms predominate, any comorbidities and the short- and long-term benefits and drawbacks of each therapy.
- For the initial management levodopa, dopamine agonists or monoamine oxidase-B (MAO-B) inhibitors are recommended.
- Second-line strategies usually involve the combination of levodopa and a dopamine agonist.
- The addition of amantadine is useful for the management of drug-induced dyskinesias.
- Catechol-O-methyltransferase (COMT) inhibitors and MAO-B inhibitors are useful for the management of end-of-dose wearing off and on/off fluctuations.
- When these strategies fail, the last lines of pharmacological therapy are apomorphine and Duodopa, a levodopa preparation that is delivered directly into the small intestine.
- Anticholinergic drugs are only rarely used owing to their adverse effects and poor efficacy. They have a small effect on early tremor but no effect on rigidity and bradykinesia.
- Symptomatic treatment should also be provided for the associated symptoms such as constipation and depression, with care to avoid drugs that may worsen the other symptoms.
- Surgery to provide deep brain stimulation may be undertaken in those who are refractory to all drug therapies.

Monitoring

- The patient's response to therapy should be reviewed by specialists regularly and action taken if there is a wearing off of response, onset of additional symptoms or adverse effects.
- Each drug treatment also has its own specific monitoring requirements.

Levodopa

- Levodopa is a biological precursor of dopamine and has useful effects in the brain but can cause adverse effects through its actions in the periphery.
- Levodopa must be given in conjunction with a peripheral dopa-decarboxylase inhibitor, either benserazide or carbidopa, to avoid its breakdown prior to crossing the blood–brain barrier. Dopa-decarboxylase inhibitors do not cross the blood–brain barrier. They also prevent some of the adverse effects of increasing dopamine in the periphery, especially nausea and hypotension.
- Levodopa is the most effective initial treatment for Parkinson's disease, with effects on bradykinesia, hypokinesia and rigidity, although the effects wear off in all patients over time.
- It is usually initiated in low doses and built up gradually to allow tolerance to adverse effects.
- Its most concerning side-effect is the production of dyskinesias, which are involuntary movements.
- It also produces 'wearing off' and 'on/off' fluctuations. These have an 'on' phase of normal movement and 'off' phase of weakness and akinesia.
- These adverse effects can be partly managed by adjusting the dose and frequency, using modified-release and dispersible preparations, or by the addition of other medications such as COMT or MAO-B inhibitors.

Dopamine agonists

- There are a number of dopamine agonists, including the ergot derivatives bromocriptine and cabergoline and the non-ergots pramipexole, ropinirole and rotigotine.
- They are available as oral preparations with the exception of rotigotine, which is available as a patch providing transdermal delivery.
- They may improve the 'on/off' fluctuations and dyskinesias with levodopa.
- Patients should be observed for the development of neuropsychiatric symptoms, such as hallucinations.
- They cause drowsiness and patients should be counselled against operating machinery or driving.

- The ergot-derived dopamine agonists may produce pulmonary fibrosis, for which monitoring by respiratory function and chest radiography should be performed.

Other drugs

- COMT inhibitors may increase the side-effects of levodopa and cause diarrhoea.
- MAO-B inhibitors may cause hypotension, falls and worsening depression, all requiring monitored.
- Amantadine has dopaminergic and antimuscarinic effects. It can produce ankle oedema, urinary retention and skin discolouration.
- Apomorphine is given via subcutaneous injection or infusion and treatment must be monitored for injection site reaction. Apomorphine is highly emetogenic and domperidone must be administered regularly for at least 2 days prior to therapy and gradually weaned off if possible.

Counselling

- A full understanding of each drug is necessary. Often, the complexity of treatment increases as the disease progresses. Compliance aids and medication summary sheets may be useful tools.
- Patients often have problems opening child-proof containers or using blister strips as they lack fine movements. Solutions to these barriers to therapy should be sought.
- All potential adverse effects should be explained and patients should be given strategies to counteract these.
- The risk of falls is increased in Parkinson's disease and counselling on avoiding falls and on other medications that may contribute to them is important.

Tip

Prescribing and dispensing errors are common with levodopa preparations. Care should always be taken to ensure that the correct product is provided and that patients are aware of how to take each.

- The possibility of drug interactions should always be borne in mind and patients should be aware of the need to check with their pharmacist or doctor prior to taking any new medication.
- Keeping a symptom diary may be useful when for decision making on adjusting therapy as it allows correlations between symptoms and adverse effects and medication administration to be made.
- Dopamine agonists and levodopa are best taken with food.
- COMT inhibitors may cause discolouration of urine.
- The dopamine agonists are associated with 'impulse control disorder'. Patients and their carers should be warned of

this disorder, which can lead to actions such as impulsive gambling, hypersexuality and aggression.

Multiple choice questions

1. **Which of the following are characteristics of Parkinson's disease?**
a. Macrographia
b. Tremor
c. Quicker than usual movements
d. Shuffling gait
e. Muscle rigidity

2. **Are the following statements true or false?**
a. The symptoms of Parkinson's disease are rapidly progressive.
b. Apomorphine is the only parenteral anti-Parkinson's drug.
c. Parkinson-like symptoms can be induced by metoclopramide.
d. MOA-A inhibitors are used in the treatment of Parkinson's disease.
e. Levodopa can cause hypotension and nausea and must be adminis-tered with a dopa-decarboxylase inhibitor.

Useful websites

www.nice.org.uk
www.parkinsons.org.uk
www.michaeljfox.org

chapter 21

Alzheimer's disease

Overview

- Alzheimer's disease has a detrimental effect on both cognitive and memory function.
- It is important to counsel patients and their carers on the disease and its treatment.
- Treatment options are limited and even those who show an initial response will eventually deteriorate.
- Compliance aids can be very useful in this group of patients.

Aetiology

- Alzheimer's disease is characterised by both cell structure and biochemical changes.
- It is associated with the presence of amyloid plaques and neurofibrillary tangles in the brain. These cause neuronal death in the cortical and subcortical regions.
- Amyloid plaques are formed by the accumulation of beta-amyloid proteins; neurofibrillary tangles result from hyperphosphorylation of tau proteins. The reasons why these occur are not understood.
- It is thought that declining memory and cognitive function results from a lack of acetylcholine and an excess of excitatory amino acids, especially glutamate.
- Acetylcholine is normally broken down by two cholinesterase enzymes, acetylcholinesterase and butyrylcholinesterase. In Alzheimer's disease, the decline in activity of acetylcholine is accompanied by a decrease in the production of acetylcholinesterase; however, there is an increase in butyrylcholinesterase, further contributing to the decline of acetylcholine levels.
- Glutamate is a major excitatory neurotransmitter. Its action on the NMDA (N-methyl-D-aspartate) receptor can lead to overstimulation of neurones, causing permanent damage.

Epidemiology

- Alzheimer's disease is the fourth leading cause of death in the Western world.
- Incidence increases with age, affecting 1% of those aged 60–65 and rising to 40% in those aged over 80 years.

Tip

Many drugs may cause confusion in the elderly, which may be mistaken for signs of Alzheimer's disease. These include anti-Parkinson drugs, benzodiazepines, diuretics, diabetic drugs, monoamine oxidase inhibitors, opioids, steroids and tricyclic antidepressants.

- Risk factors proposed include:
  - increasing age
  - female
  - family history
  - head injury
  - Parkinson's disease
  - hypothyroidism
  - chronic exposure to aluminium
  - cardiovascular disease
  - smoking
  - chronic high alcohol intake.
- Average survival time from diagnosis is 10 years, although patients and their families and carers often experience a significant decrease in quality of life for a large part of this time.

Signs and symptoms

Alzheimer's disease is characterised by a gradual decline in cognitive and memory function. This can present in a wide variety of ways, although there are few, if any, physical signs:

- unable to perform daily activities, such as dressing, washing, feeding
- behavioural problems
- reduced muscular function
- sleeplessness
- aggression
- apathy
- delusions and hallucinations
- loss of autonomic control.

Investigations

- As the condition predominately affects cognitive and memory functions, the investigations focus on these areas rather than physical examinations.
- It is only possible to make a presumed diagnosis of Alzheimer's disease, as a definite diagnosis is only possible through autopsy.
- A number of assessment methods can be utilised that define both cognitive and memory function. This includes Mini Mental State Examination (MMSE), Alzheimer's disease Assessment Scale (ADAS) and the Blessed test of information.
- Neuroimaging, using techniques such as MRI and CT, can demonstrate degenerative changes in the brain.
- It is thought that a diagnosis can be made with approximately 80–90% accuracy using these methods.

Management

- The aim of treatment is to relieve symptoms and prevent the progression of the disease.
- Four drugs are currently available in the UK for the treatment of Alzheimer's disease: the cholinesterase inhibitors donepezil, galantamine and rivastigmine and the NMDA receptor antagonist memantine.
- They can only be initiated by specialists in the care of patients with Alzheimer's disease.
- The cholinesterase inhibitors act by increasing the amount of acetylcholine available at the synaptic junction. Galantamine has also some additional activity as an agonist at acetylcholine nicotinic receptors.
- Approximately 30–50% of patients show a definable decrease in their rate of cognitive decline after 3 months of treatment.
- The main adverse effects are from their cholinergic activity, such as nausea, vomiting, diarrhoea, anorexia, urinary frequency and depression. This can be a problem as those with Alzheimer's disease are often at risk of losing weight through the disease.
- To decrease the potential side-effects, the drugs are introduced gradually with a steady dose titration.
- There is no evidence for chosing one cholinesterase inhibitor rather than another. Only donepezil and modified-release galantamine can be taken once daily.
- Memantine is licensed for the treatment of moderate to severe disease but is only recommended to be used in the UK as part of clinical studies, as there is a lack of comparative date with the other therapies.
- Atypical antipsychotic drugs and haloperidol are sometimes used to manage the behavioural problems that can occur in Alzheimer's.

Tips

Anxiolytics are often prescribed to manage the symptoms of Alzheimer's disease but may contribute to an increase in confusion and the risk of falls.
  Other drugs that have been used in the treatment of Alzheimer's disease include *Gingko biloba*, vitamin E, selegiline, oestrogens and physostigmine.

Monitoring parameters

- As the response rates to Alzheimer's treatment are relatively low and the drugs are costly, their efficacy must be reviewed regularly in all patients.
- It is recommended that patients are reviewed for benefit after 2 to 4 months after reaching the recommended maintenance dose. If benefit is not demonstrated, the drugs should be stopped.
- Even those who show an initial response will eventually stop gaining benefit from treatment, and at this stage their treatment

should be discontinued; this point is often defined as a MMSE score of 10.

■ Assessment for efficacy utilises the same assessment tools as for diagnosis.

■ Patients should also be monitored for adverse effects.

Counselling

■ An attempt should be made to educate the patient regarding their disease and drug therapy; however, in Alzheimer's disease it is often a patient's carer who will be responsible for the treatment. Verbal and written information should be given to both parties.

Tip

Weight loss can be a problem in Alzheimer's disease, from both the condition itself and the medication used to treat it. Advice on appropriate dietary intake should be provided.

■ Compliance aids are often useful for this group of patients, as they often have other conditions requiring medications owing to their age group.

■ Pharmacists can also help to promote awareness of non-drug therapies such as cognitive–behavioural therapy and occupational therapy.

■ Patients and their carers should be aware of the potential side-effects of the drug therapy and how these may be managed.

Multiple choice questions

1. Which of the following is *not* licensed for the treatment of Alzheimer's disease?
a. Amantadine
b. Galantamine
c. Donepezil
d. Memantine
e. Rivastigmine

2. Are the following statements true or false?
a. All cholinesterase inhibitors must be given in divided daily doses.
b. Alzheimer's disease is caused by overactivity of acetylcholine.
c. Galantamine can cause depression, diarrhoea and nausea.
d. Memantine is *not* recommended for first-line treatment.
e. Cholinesterase inhibitors are recommended for the treatment of end-stage Alzheimer's disease.

Useful websites

www.nice.org.uk
www.alzheimers.org.uk

chapter 22

Depression

Overview

- Depression is the most common mental illness in the world.
- It is thought to be mainly a result of disturbances in the neurotransmitters noradrenaline and serotonin.
- Antidepressant drug therapy is recommended for those with moderate to severe disease, and those with mild disease who fail to respond to non-pharmacological measures.
- For most patients, the initial antidepressant of choice is a selective serotonin reuptake inhibitor.

Aetiology

- As is the case with other mental illness, the mechanism for the development of depression is not fully understood.
- It is thought to result from changes in the balance of neurotransmitters in certain areas of the brain and changes in receptor sensitivity.
- The two most important neurotransmitters are considered to be noradrenaline and serotonin. Deficiencies in the levels and activity of these neurotransmitters are thought to be the main cause of depression.
- Other contributing factors are thought to include hormonal imbalances affecting the hypothalamic–pituitary–adrenal axis.

Epidemiology

- Depression is the third leading cause of illness worldwide according to the World Heath Organization (WHO).
- Depression is the most common form of mental illness in the UK.
- One in five people in the UK will suffer from depression during their lifetime.
- Women are twice as likely as men to be diagnosed with depression.
- It is thought that at any one time 5–10% of the UK population is suffering from depression.
- The most likely age group to experience depression is those in their mid-20s.

Tip

Many medications may cause depression but it is not often recognised as patients make healthcare professionals aware of their depressive symptoms. Questions pertaining to the presence of new onset of depression should be included when assessing a patient's response to drug therapy with any agent known to cause depression. Examples include many commonly used drugs, such as statins, beta-blockers, oestrogens, corticosteroids and levothyroxine.

- Causes are thought to include:
  - genetic predisposition
  - emotional triggers such as trauma or bad life event
  - physical causes, e.g. comorbidities such as multiple sclerosis and cancer
  - medications, e.g. isotretinoin and interferon alfa.

Signs and symptoms

As with other forms of mental illness, the signs and symptoms are manifested in emotional ways rather than in an openly physical manner. The main symptoms are low mood or loss of interest, accompanied by one or more of:

- fatigue
- changes in appetite or weight
- sleep disturbances
- poor concentration
- feelings of guilt or worthlessness
- suicidal ideas.

Investigations

Tip

Questioning patients who may have depression should aim to assess both the presence and the frequency of symptoms and their effect on the patient. Suggested questions include 'During the last month, have you felt down, depressed or hopeless?' and 'During the last month, how often have you been bothered by having little interest or pleasure in doing things?'

- Those who should be investigated for the presence of depression include:
  - those presenting with symptoms of depression
  - those with a history of depression
  - those with significant physical illnesses causing disability
  - those with other mental health illnesses, such as dementia.
- Potential physical or medication causes should be assessed.
- Assessment is made using screening questions to assess severity of symptoms.
- Validated assessment tools are widely used to assess depression symptom severity and general well-being; these include the WHO *International Classification of Diseases*.[1]
- Physical examination may be necessary prior to starting antidepressant therapy. The type of investigations depends on the drug therapy choice and the patient's medical history.

Management

- The goals of treatment in depression are to attempt to cure the illness and to provide relief of symptoms, while minimising the risk of adverse effects.

- Management of depression follows a stepwise approach depending on the severity of symptoms and the degree of specialism of treatment provision. There are 5 steps:

Step 1 is the initial assessment of depression and does not involve initiation of treatment

Step 2 is the initiation of appropriate therapy for mild depression in primary care

Step 3 is the management of moderate to severe depression in primary care

Step 4 is the treatment of severe or unresponsive depression by mental health specialists

Step 5 is the inpatient management of depression by mental health specialists.

- The majority of patients are managed through steps 1 and 2, with the numbers at each step from 1 to 5 decreasing.
- Each step involves the utilisation of a number of treatment strategies. The merit of each option should be discussed fully with the patient and a joint decision on which therapy to use should be made.

Step 2: mild depression

Regardless of the therapy chosen, all patients should receive review to determine whether symptoms are improving or deteriorating. Options for those with mild depression include:

- watchful waiting, where the patient decides not to receive treatment or may recover without intervention; they should be reviewed after 2 months to determine whether treatment is needed
- exercise programmes, consisting of up to three supervised sessions per week of 45–60 min over a 10–12 week period
- sleep and anxiety management techniques
- guided self-help, involving the provision of limited supported and written materials for 6 to 9 weeks
- computer-based cognitive–behavioural therapy
- psychological therapy.

Antidepressants are not recommended for initial therapy in mild depression as the risks outweigh the benefits. They may be considered in:

- those where other interventions fail
- those who have depression associated with medical problems
- those who currently have mild depression but have a history of moderate to severe depression.

Step 3: moderate to severe depression

Antidepressants are indicated in those with moderate or severe depression. They may be used in conjunction with other management techniques, such as those used in mild depression.

Steps 4 and 5: severe or unresponsive depression

- Management is by specialists in mental health and includes intensive psychological methods, combinations of drug therapy and the use of electroconvulsive therapy (ECT).
- Selective serotonin reuptake inhibitors (SSRIs) are considered first-line antidepressant therapy because of their similar efficacy but superior tolerability and safety when compared with tricyclic antidepressants.
- Fluoxetine and citalopram are the most commonly used SSRIs as they are available as generic preparations and are thought to have fewer withdrawal symptoms than paroxetine.
- Sertraline is the usual drug of choice in those with unstable angina or previous myocardial infarction, based on evidence for its use in these patients.
- Patients failing to respond to an SSRI should try another SSRI or mirtazepine, a serotonin–noradrenaline reuptake inhibitor (SNRI).
- Tricyclic antidepressants, such as lofepramine and amitriptyline, are another second-line option in some patients.
- Monoamine oxidase (MAO) inhibitors and venlafaxine (SNRI) are used by specialists for those with unresponsive disease.
- In those failing to response to two different agents, a combination of antidepressants with different modes of action may be trialed by specialists.
- The presence of comorbidities and other drug therapies should always be considered when making a choice of antidepressant.

Monitoring parameters

- All those starting antidepressant therapy should be reviewed every 1–2 weeks.
- Antidepressants take at least 4 weeks to have a significant effect, so a decision on effectiveness should not be taken until at least this time.
- The dose of antidepressant may be increased at this time if there has been a partial response.
- Patients should be monitored every 2–4 weeks for the first 3 months and then at regular intervals.
- Patients should also be monitored for the presence of adverse effects regularly and therapy changed if any significant adverse effects arise.
- Treatment should continue for at least 6 months after remission for all patients and for 2 years in those with a history of recurrent depression.

- Sudden cessation of therapy may be possible in some patients; however, many will suffer withdrawal symptoms. These include GI disturbances, headache, anorexia, panic, anxiety and restlessness.
- If this occurs, therapy should be withdrawn gradually over periods of 1 to 6 months.
- Specific monitoring is required for each therapy and may be influenced by any comorbidity present in the patient.
- All antidepressants have been associated with hyponatraemia as a result of inappropriate antidiuretic hormone secretion. This is more common with SSRIs than other antidepressants.

Selective serotonin reuptake inhibitors
- SSRIs are generally well tolerated; however, they may commonly cause GI effects, including nausea, vomiting, dyspepsia, diarrhoea or constipation, as well as anorexia, rash, arthralgia and hypotension.
- They have been linked with suicidal tendencies, especially upon initiation and in children. Patients and their carers should be aware of this and monitored for its occurrence at each review.
- SSRIs may increase the risk for gastric bleeding. Patients should monitor for signs of this, especially those also taking NSAIDs, antiplatelet drugs or anticoagulants.

Tricyclic antidepressants
- The most common adverse effects with tricyclic antidepressants are related to their antimuscarinic activity, such as dry mouth, drowsiness, blurred vision, urinary retention, constipation and sweating.
- Tolerance to these adverse effects may occur, especially if low starting doses and gradual titration is used.
- Tricyclic antidepressants are associated with cardiac arrhythmias and heart block, especially in those with cardiac disease. Such patients should receive an ECG prior to therapy and blood pressure monitoring at each review.
- Lofepramine is considered the safest in patients with cardiac disease.

Serotonin–noradrenaline reuptake inhibitors
- SRNIs have similar adverse effects to SSRIs but generally have few antimuscarinic effects.
- Mirtazepine is associated with blood dyscrasias. Patients should seek medical attention if signs of these occur. It may also cause weight gain and sedation.
- Venlafaxine is often poorly tolerated and its adverse effects are common. In addition, patients should receive regular blood pressure monitoring and an ECG prior to therapy if they have cardiac disease.

Tip

St John's wort is one of the most commonly taken herbal medications in the UK and often used for the treatment of depression, often self-diagnosed. It is not known whether it is as efficacious as conventional therapies. It has many interactions with other medications as it induces cytochrome P450 isoenzymes, for example warfarin, digoxin, antiretroviral drugs, theophylline, oestrogen and ciclosporin.

Monoamine oxidase inhibitors

- MAO inhibitors may cause accumulation of amine neurotransmitters, leading to dangerous rises in blood pressure.
- They have many drug interactions, especially with other antidepressants.
- They are prescribed only by specialists.
- They can interact with tyramine-rich foods such as mature cheese, broad beans, yeast extracts and stale foods.

Counselling

- Patients should be made aware that the effects of antidepressants can take up to 4 weeks to become apparent.
- Patients should understand that antidepressants must be taken regularly to have effect and that withdrawal symptoms may occur on discontinuation.
- Those withdrawing from therapy should report any withdrawal effects and be given a personalised regimen for withdrawal if it is a problem.

Tip

Antidepressants have a relatively poor success rate, with only around half of patients responding to each agent. Patients should be aware of this prior to therapy and be supported through the acute phase.

- Patients should be aware of other potential adverse effects and that their medications may interact with many others.
- Patients on all antidepressants, especially SSRIs, should be aware of the signs of hyponatraemia, such as confusion, drowsiness and convulsion, and seek urgent medical attention if they develop.
- Patients on mirtazepine should seek urgent medical attention if they have signs of blood dyscrasias such as sore throat, fever, stomatitis or infection.
- Patients taking tricyclic antidepressants should be aware of their potential antimuscarinic effects and be given support to minimise these effects, such as laxatives for constipation.
- Tricyclic antidepressants cause sedation so are best taken at night to minimise associated risks. This side-effect may also be beneficial in those with sleep disturbances.

Multiple choice questions

1. Which of the following does *not* interact with St John's wort?
a. Digoxin
b. Warfarin

c. Theophylline
d. Erythromycin
e. Combined oral contraceptive pill

2. **Are the following statements true or false?**
a. Lofepramine is the tricyclic antidepressant of choice in those with cardiac disease.
b. SSRIs are the first-line treatment for those presenting with mild depression.
c. Initial antidepressant should be changed in those with a partial response after 4 weeks.
d. SSRIs may cause gastric bleeding.
e. Antidepressant therapy should be continued for 6 months after resolution of symptoms.

Reference

1. World Health Organization (1992). *International Classification of Diseases and Problems*, 10th edn. Geneva: World Health Organization.

Useful website

www.nice.org.uk

chapter 23

Schizophrenia

Overview

- The pathology causing schizophrenia is not yet fully understood.
- A large number of agents can be used in its management; these are broadly classed as typical or atypical antipsychotics.
- All treatments are associated with potentially serious side-effects.
- Treatment must be carefully tailored to the individual patient.
- Therapy must normally be continued for at least 2 years in all patients.

Aetiology

- The pathology of schizophrenia is poorly understood.
- It is thought of as a neurodevelopmental condition rather than a neurodegenerative disorder, such as Parkinson's or Alzheimer's disease.
- Classically, it has been thought that the main pathology was linked to overactivity of the dopaminergic neurotransmission. As such, traditional therapies have consisted of dopamine receptor antagonists, for example chlorpromazine.
- The lack of an immediate response to dopamine receptor antagonists indicates that there are other processes involved.
- At present it is postulated that changes in the number of receptors expressed in cells or alterations in intracellular signal transduction may play a part in the condition.
- In addition to targeting the dopaminergic system, currently utilised drug therapy also acts on serotonergic, glutamatergic, GABAergic and noradrenergic systems.
- Drugs acting on NMDA receptors, such as ketamine, can lead to schizophrenia-like symptoms so these may also play a role.

Epidemiology

- Schizophrenia is thought to affect 20 million people worldwide, with half of these being in the developed world.
- It is estimated to affect 1% of the UK population.
- The age of onset is commonly during a patient's early 20s.

Tip

Schizophrenia is poorly understood by the general public; therefore, diagnosis may be delayed and patients may be stigmatised. It is important not to make any assumptions about patients and treat them all with empathy.

- Up to 20% of patients suffer only a single acute episode.
- The cause of death in appropriately 10% of those with schizophrenia is suicide.
- Drug use, such as amphetamines, is responsible for some cases; however, other risk factors have yet to be well defined.

Signs and symptoms

An acute episode can be divided into positive and negative symptoms:

- *positive symptoms*
- hallucinations, such as perceived sounds, images, tastes, smells or other sensory experiences without a real stimulus
- thought disorders and disorganised communication, such as thought broadcasting where the sufferer thinks that others can read their thoughts
- delusions, which may present as irrational beliefs
- *negative symptoms*
- withdrawing from social contact
- reduced activity accompanied by emotional flattening
- mood abnormality, such as anxiety, depression or irritability
- cognitive impairment, such as poverty of thought.
- Patients may have some or all of the symptoms during an acute episode, with some being more prominent than others; for example, in some patients thought disorders may dominate whereas in others it may be delusions.
- Chronically, schizophrenic patients may have a course of relapses involving acute symptoms but overall will often develop social withdrawal and apathy.
- Negative symptoms are often much more difficult to treat than positive symptoms.

> **Tip**
>
> The term schizophrenia comes from the Greek words *skhizo* meaning to split and *phren* meaning mind. It represents the splitting of intellect and emotion, not split personalities.

Investigations

- Making a diagnosis of schizophrenia is difficult as there are few objective measurements possible.
- The criteria laid out in the American Psychiatric Association's *Diagnostic and Statistical Manual of Mental Disorders* are usually used to reach a diagnosis.[1] These state that a patient must have at least two of the following symptoms present the majority of the time over a month:
- delusions
- hallucinations
- disorganised speech
- disorganised or catatonic behaviour

— negative symptoms, such as emotional flattening.
- A diagnosis is also made if a patient's symptoms improve on receiving antipsychotic therapy.
- In patients with mild, persistent symptoms, a diagnosis may take 6 months or more.
- It is important to ensure there are no other causes such as substance abuse or physical change (e.g. brain tumours).

Management

- Drugs used for the management of schizophrenia can be broadly split into two categories; typical and atypical antipsychotics.
- Both classes have a significant action on dopamine D_2 receptors.
- Current treatment strategies, including NICE guidance, recommend that the newer atypical antipsychotic drugs should be use as the initial treatment, as they have less association with the development of extrapyramidal effects.
- The aims of treatment are to:
— manage initial psychotic symptoms
— improve quality of life
— attempt to prevent relapse
— avoid or minimise adverse effects.
- Extrapyramidal and endocrine symptoms can be a problem in many patients, especially when reaching higher doses.
- Inhibition of dopamine transmission can cause hyperprolactinaemia.
- The differences in the effects of individual drugs mainly reflect their relative actions on α-adrenoceptors and histamine, muscarinic and serotonin receptors.
- Treatment is often long term. As a minimum, patients who have experienced only one acute episode in the preceding 1 to 2 years and appear to be in remission can have their medication gradually withdrawn and should then be monitored for the return of symptoms for at least 2 years after their last episode.
- Those who have experienced two or more acute episodes should receive at least 5 years of therapy before an attempt is made to withdraw treatment.

Atypical antipsychotic drugs
- Atypical antipsychotic drugs include olanzapine, quetiapine, risperidone and zotepine.
- They have differing side-effect profiles, cautions, formulations and dosing schedules, and careful consideration must be given to which is the appropriate agent for each patient.
- They are associated with weight gain and metabolic disorders, such as diabetes.

- *Clozapine* is an atypical antipsychotic drug that is not recommended as first-line therapy. It is often effective in those who have an inadequate response to other antipsychotic drugs and is especially active against negative symptoms. It should only be used in those with treatment-resistant schizophrenia who have tried at least two antipsychotic drugs, at least one of which was atypical, at recommended doses for 6–8 weeks. This is because there is a drug-specific risk of agranulocytosis. Patients initiated on clozapine require specific, intense monitoring.

Tip

In addition to oral preparations, there are a number of 'depot' injection preparations. These are administered at intervals of 1 to 4 weeks and are particularly beneficial in those with compliance problems. Where possible, patients should receive the drug in oral test doses to ensure they tolerate it, as any side-effects experienced after depot injection will be long lasting.

Typical antipsychotic drugs

- The largest group in the typical antipsychotic class is the phenothiazines. These are split into three groups according to their structure:
  - group 1 (aliphatic), e.g. chlorpromazine, levomepromazine
  - group 2 (piperidine), e.g. thioridazine
  - group 3 (piperazine), e.g. prochlorperazine and trifluoperazine.
- Others in the typical antipsychotic class are similar in structure to group 3 phenothiazines and include the butylophenones (e.g. haloperidol), thioxanthines (e.g. flupentixol) and substituted benzamides (e.g. sulpiride).
- The typical antipsychotic drugs are associated with side-effects such as extrapyramidal effects, hypotension and antimuscarinic effects.

Tip

The atypical drugs were initially thought to have relatively few significant side-effects compared with the typical group; however, their propensity to cause weight gain and diabetes has led to an increase in the use of the typical antipsychotic drugs in many patients.

Monitoring parameters

- Patients must be regularly monitored for both efficacy and adverse effects.
- Efficacy is assessed through measurement of the presence and severity of the initial symptoms, and ensuring that no new symptoms have developed.
- Monitoring of adverse effects is dependent on the individual drug, but in general will include baseline and follow-up assessment of blood pressure, ECG to detect any conduction abnormalities, weight, urinary and blood glucose, and liver and kidney function tests.
- Temperature may be assessed as an early diagnostic tool for the development of the rare but potentially serious neuroleptic malignant syndrome.

- Common adverse effects and the drugs they are most associated with include:
- — weight gain with atypical drugs
- — sexual dysfunction with sulpiride
- — endocrine effects, such as galactorrhoea and amenorrhoea with sulpiride and phenothiazines
- — extrapyramidal effects with haloperidol and the phenothiazines
- — antimuscarinic effects with clozapine and phenothiazines
- — cardiac arrhythmias with sertindole, phenothiazines, clozapine
- — blood dyscrasias with clozapine
- — hypotension with quetiapine, haloperidol, phenothiazines
- — drowsiness with chlorpromazine.

Counselling

- Patients and their carers should be fully aware of the disease and the medication being used.
- Patients may lack insight into their condition and have a distrust of people, both of which may change during therapy so important information should be reinforced at available opportunities.
- Any possible side-effects should be explained fully in advance of therapy to reduce the risk of non-compliance.
- Potentially serious side-effects should be emphasised, such as the risk of agranulocytosis with clozapine. Patients taking a drug should be clear on the signs of the adverse effect, such as sore throat and temperature.
- Supportive care for some side-effects may be provided, such as laxatives and artificial saliva for antimuscarinic effects.
- Lifestyle and healthy eating advice should be provided in an attempt to minimise potential weight gain and risk of diabetes and associated cardiac problems.

Multiple choice questions

1. Which of the following is *not* a potential adverse effect of phenothiazine type of antipsychotic drug?
a. Hypotension
b. Excessive saliva
c. Extrapyramidal effects
d. Sexual dysfunction
e. Galactorrhoea

2. Are the following statements true or false?
a. All schizophrenia patients will suffer from hallucinations.
b. Quetiapine is associated with agranulocytosis.
c. Olanzapine is an atypical antipsychotic drug.

d. Patients must have received at least three different antipsychotic drugs prior to a trial of clozapine.

e. Thought disorders are considered negative symptoms.

Reference

1. American Psychiatric Association, (1995). *Diagnostic and Statistical Manual of Mental Disorders*, 4th edn. Washington, DC: American Psychiatric Press.

Useful website

www.nice.org.uk

Overview

- Pain is always subjective and management differs for different patients.
- Acute pain is transient and lasts for no more than 2–3 days.
- Chronic pain is persistent pain and is more a disease than a symptom.
- Pain can be somatic, visceral or neuropathic.

Aetiology

- Pain can be acute or chronic.
- Acute pain is mediated by adrenaline. It is transient, lasting for no more than 2 to 3 days.
- Chronic pain is persistent and has been described as more of a disease than a symptom.
- Pain is subjective: the patient knows best of how much pain they are feeling.
- There are three main types of pain:
- somatic pain originates from the nociceptors in deep tissue (e.g. bone, muscles, joints); it is a sharp localised pain, often described as a gnawing or aching pain
- visceral pain originates from the nociceptors in the throrax, abdomen and pelvis; it is a deep, unlocalised pain, often constant and diffused
- neuropathic pain originates from the CNS; it is described as burning, constricting, paroxysmal or shooting.

Defining pain

The 'standard' definition of pain is that of the International Association for the Study of Pain: 'An unpleasant sensory or emotional experience associated with actual or potential tissue damage, or described in terms of such damage. Pain is always subjective. Each individual learns the application of the word through experiences related to injury in early life. It is unquestionably a sensation in a part of the body, but it is also unpleasant, and therefore also an emotional experience. Many people report pain in the absence of tissue damage or any likely pathophysiological cause; usually this happens for psychological reasons. There is no way to distinguish their experience from that due to tissue damage, if we take this subjective report.'

Investigations: assessment of pain

- Thorough consultation with the patient is required.
- A full analgesic history is taken.
- The patient's own description of pain will include:
- detailed history of the site, intensity, frequency, radiation, timing, quality of pain
- factors that aggravate or relieve the pain.
- Level of pain can be gauged using visual analogue scales and pain questionnaires.
- Diagnostic tests such as radiography and imaging techniques are used where required.

Management

- The WHO analgesic ladder provides a stepwise approach to the treatment of somatic and visceral pain (Table 24.1).[1]

Tip

If treatment with a weak opioid is ineffective, it is best to step up treatment as nothing is gained by substituting with another weak opioid.

- Treatment aims to achieve freedom from pain:
- at night to allow sleep
- during day at rest
- on movement.
- Pain medication should be taken at regular intervals.
- Other interventions can be used to bring patients down a step on the analgesic ladder.
- Patients can move up or down a step depending on their pain control; regular review is, therefore, recommended.
- Moderate pain is treated with weak opioids, e.g. codeine, dihydrocodeine
- paracetamol can be continued as it has synergistic action
- co-dydramol and co-proxamol are prescribed to simplify regimens.
- Neuropathic pain is treated with adjuvant drugs; these have no intrinsic analgesic properties but will relieve pain in this circumstance.

Table 24.1 A stepwise approach to analgesia

Stage	Treatment	Examples
Rung 1	Non-opioids ± adjuvants	Paracetamol, NSAIDs
Rung 2	Opioids of weak potency plus non-opioids ± adjuvants	Codeine, dihydrocodeine, tramadol
Rung 3	Opioids of strong potency	Morphine, fentanyl, methadone, hydromorphone

Adjuvants: carbamazepine, steroids, biphosphonates.
Based on World Health Organization. *Cancer Pain Relief and Palliative Care.*[1]

Monitoring parameters: analgesic drugs

Table 24.2 gives the medications available, their actions and side-effects.

Table 24.2 Analgesic drugs

Name or class of analgesic	Mode of action	Side-effects	Any other information
Paracetamol	Thought to act centrally, but not well understood	Side-effects are rare; rashes and blood disorders have been reported	Maximum 4 g in 24 h; patient should not take any other paracetamol-containing products
NSAIDs, e.g. ibuprofen, naproxen	Inhibit COX-1 and COX-2, which synthesise prostaglandins; prostaglandins are responsible for pain, inflammation and fever and also protect the stomach lining	GI bleeding, nausea, vomiting, diarrhoea, rash, hypersensitivity, renal failure, hepatic failure	Suitable for the relief of toothache, dysmenorrhoea and joint pain. Can be used as an adjuvant at any step of the ladder
COX-2 inhibitors, e.g. celecoxib	Inhibit COX-2 only	Nausea, vomiting, abdominal pain, cardiotoxicity	GI side-effects less than with NSAIDs
Opioids	Bind to specific receptors in brain and spinal cord; can be full or partial agonists or antagonists. Three different subtypes of receptors; most strong opioids are strong μ (mu) agonists	Reduced GI motility, anticholinergic side-effects (dry mouth, blurred vision, urinary retention, drowsiness and constipation), nausea and vomiting. Respiratory depression (potentially life threatening)	Tolerance to side-effects often occurs. If patient is taking regular opioids, antiemetics and laxatives should be co-prescribed (usually only with the strong opioids)
Codeine	Structurally similar to morphine		Potent cough suppressant, short duration of action
Morphine	Works throughout the CNS		Variety of short/long-acting solid and liquid formulations; diamorphine preferred for SC infusion. Opioid toxicity may occur (respiratory depression); naloxone (opioid antagonist) can reverse this effect

Table 24.2 (continued)

Fentanyl	Synthetic opioid with rapid onset and short duration of action if given IV; metabolised in the liver. Transdermal application avoids first-pass effect and creates depot in skin. Has low molecular weight, high solubility and long half life; steady-state plasma concentration achieved within 36–48 h; elimination half life ≥17 h. Care when changing from IV/oral to transdermal. Can take up to 72 h for depot to clear
Hydromorphone	Controlled-release and immediate-release formulations available. Seven times more potent than morphine with fewer side-effects. Patients experiencing confusion, hallucinations, vivid dreams, loss of concentration with morphine may benefit if use hydromorphone

COX, cyclo-oxygenase.

Overall approach to pain management

- The patient should be carefully assessed for their pain, with a full history of the pain and full medical and drug history.
- Assessment tools such as the pain questionnaire should be used to monitor the pain.
- Drugs to alleviate and control the pain should be prescribed based on the WHO analgesic ladder, a stepwise approach.
- Patients can be moved up or down the step depending on their response to pain; regular pain reviews are required especially for chronic pain such as pain in palliative care.
- Side-effects of analgesics should be carefully explained, and where possible drugs should be prescribed to treat the side-effects. For example, in the case of morphine and other strong opioids, antiemetics and laxatives should be prescribed.

Multiple choice questions

1. Which of the following is *not* a side-effect of opioids?
a. Drowsiness
b. Muscle weakness
c. Dry mouth
d. Constipation
e. Vomiting

2. Are the following statements true or false?
a. Hydromorphone is a weak opioid.
b. Pain can be of a somatic origin.
c. Gabapentin is an adjuvant used for neuropathic pain.
d. Pain is subjective to the patient.

Reference

1. World Health Organization, (1990). *Cancer Pain Relief and Palliative Care*. Geneva: World Health Organization, 1–75.

Useful websites

http://www.nhsdirect.nhs.uk
http://www.medicinenet.com/

The endocrine system

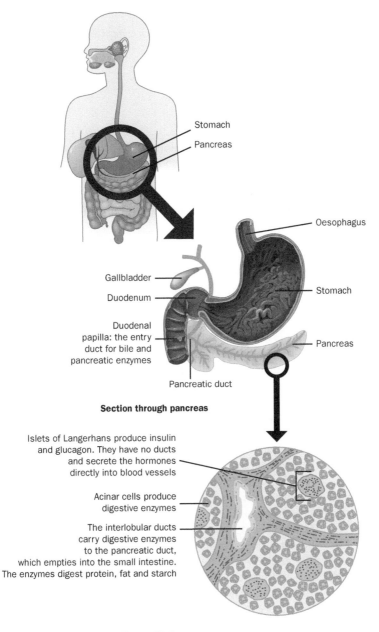

Stomach

Pancreas

Oesophagus

Gallbladder

Duodenum

Stomach

Duodenal papilla: the entry duct for bile and pancreatic enzymes

Pancreas

Pancreatic duct

Section through pancreas

Islets of Langerhans produce insulin and glucagon. They have no ducts and secrete the hormones directly into blood vessels

Acinar cells produce digestive enzymes

The interlobular ducts carry digestive enzymes to the pancreatic duct, which empties into the small intestine. The enzymes digest protein, fat and starch

Figure 25.1

Overview

- Diabetes mellitus is most common endocrine disorder in the UK.
- It is characterised by impairment of glucose metabolism.
- There are two main types, type 1 and type 2, relating to the underlying cause.
- Insulin is required for all type 1 diabetics.
- Type 2 diabetics may be managed with combinations involving oral glycaemics, diet and sometimes insulin.
- Diabetes can lead to microvascular and macrovascular complications and is a large risk factor in the development of cardiovascular disease.

Aetiology

- Diabetes mellitus is an endocrine disorder characterised by impairment in glucose metabolism.
- There are two main types of diabetes: type 1 and type 2.
- Type 1 diabetes, formerly known as insulin-dependent diabetes mellitus (IDDM), is caused by destruction of the insulin-producing beta-cells of the pancreas.
- This loss of beta-cells usually results from autoimmune-mediated destruction by T-cells or from idiopathic causes.
- In type 1 diabetes, there is a lack of insulin, which leads to hepatic glycogenolysis and gluconeogenesis and reduced uptake of glucose in insulin-sensitive tissues and causes hypoglycaemia.
- Type 2 diabetes, formerly known as non-insulin-dependent diabetes mellitus (NIDDM), results from lack of sufficient insulin production and/or lack of sensitivity to the effects of insulin. This is sometimes termed 'insulin resistance'.
- The process of development of type 2 diabetes is much slower, with a number of mechanisms involved, such as increased insulin production in response to decreased tissue insulin sensitivity. However, it eventually leads to beta-cell destruction and lack of endogenous insulin production.
- Diabetes can lead to long-term complications. These can be classified as microvascular and macrovascular.
- Microvascular complications include nephropathy, peripheral neuropathy and retinopathy.
- Macrovascular complications include peripheral vascular disease and cardiovascular diseases, such as stroke and myocardial infarction.
- Both microvascular and macrovascular changes are involved in the production of diabetic foot ulcers. Diabetic patients are 15 times more likely to have a lower limb amputated than the general population.

Epidemiology

- Diabetes is the most commonly occurring endocrine disease in the UK, with approximately 2.3 million people diagnosed with the condition and up to 1 million who have yet to be diagnosed.
- Type 1 diabetes is less common than type 2, accounting for 10–15% of diabetes diagnosis.
- Both types are becoming increasingly common worldwide.
- There is a strong genetic link in type 1 diabetes. It is more common in some ethnic groups than others, with a high incidence in Caucasians, but very low in Japanese.
- Type 1 has a younger onset than type 2, with most cases diagnosed in those under 40 years, and half in those under 20 years.
- There is also a genetic link in the development of type 2 diabetes.
- Type 2 diabetes is usually associated with obesity and often presents in association with hypertension, dyslipidaemias and cardiovascular disease.

> **Tip**
>
> Type 2 diabetes is classed as part of the much debated 'metabolic syndrome' or 'diabesity'. Other aspects of this condition include hypertension, central obesity, dyslipidaemias and atherosclerosis. The existence of this entity is not accepted by all but the term is becoming more commonly used for the presence of these risk factors.

Signs and symptoms

- The predominant symptoms of both types 1 and 2 diabetes are the same:
- increased thirst
- increased micturition (polyuria)
- nocturia
- glycosuria
- fatigue
- increase in superficial infections, such as urinary-tract infections and vaginal thrush
- blurred vision
- weight loss in type 1 diabetes.
- In those with type 1 diabetes, the signs and symptoms are usually more obvious and develop over a shorter time period, usually only a few weeks.
- Approximately a third of those with type 1 diabetes present with diabetic ketoacidosis (DKA), a life-threatening disorder. Dehydration is caused by the diuresis and vomiting which occurs as the body tries to lower the high blood levels of glucose and ketones. This leads to further vomiting, blurred vision, confusion, dizziness, ketones in the breath (smelling like pear drops) and, eventually, coma and possible death.

Investigations

- Diagnosis is usually made using the WHO criteria for diagnosing diabetes. They include:
- diabetes symptoms, e.g. polyuria, unexplained weight loss, plus
- a random plasma glucose level ≥11.1 mmol/L, or
- a fasting plasma glucose level of 7.0 mmol/L, or
- a plasma glucose level ≥11.1 mmol/L 2 h after ingestion of 75 g anhydrous glucose in a glucose tolerance test.
- Single finger prick, glycosuria or glycated haemoglobin (HbA1c) results are not recommended to make a diagnosis.
- Investigations should also examine if there is any comorbidity such as hypertension and dyslipidaemia.
- The patient should also be investigated to determine if there are any secondary complications present, using renal function tests, eyesight tests and foot inspection.

Management

The aim of therapy is to manage the symptoms of diabetes, reduce the risk of secondary complications and avoid episodes of acute hyper- and hypoglycaemia.

Type 1 diabetes

- Patients with type 1 diabetes require the administration of exogenous insulin to manage their condition.
- There are many types of insulin available and injection forms. An attempt must be made to tailor the regimen to the patient's usual lifestyle and their preferences.
- It is often difficult to achieve the correct balance between tight glycaemic control and avoidance of hypoglycaemic episodes.
- Insulins may be classified as fast, intermediate and long acting, reflecting their onset and durations of action.
- The serum concentration of short-acting insulins peaks at approximately 2 h after administration, in a similar manner to endogenous insulin. They are administered prior to meals, with non-analogue forms being given 30 min prior to meals and newer analogue types, such as insulin lispro or aspart, being given as a meal is commenced.
- Intermediate-acting insulins, such as isophane or lente insulin, achieve peak concentrations approximately 4–8 h after administration and usually require twice daily dosing.
- Long-acting insulins, such as glargine and detemir insulins, have duration of activity of approximately 24 h and may be given once daily.

- Insulin regimens in type 1 diabetes require numerous injections throughout the day.
- Two regimens are commonly used: basal-bolus and twice daily.
- Basal-bolus regimens involve the administration of fast-acting insulin prior to meals and once or twice daily injections of long- or intermediate-acting insulins. This provides a pattern of insulin delivery similar to that in normal individuals.
- Twice daily injections of pre-mixed preparations of short- and intermediate-acting insulins provide a convenient compromise in many patients.
- Currently insulin is only available in injectable forms. An inhaled form was released a number of years ago but has been discontinued by its manufacturer for commercial reasons. Patients using this device still required injections of intermediate- or long-acting insulin as it was only able to deliver doses of short-acting insulin.

Type 2 diabetes
- Treatment is aimed at achieving an HbA1c between 6.5% and 7.5%.
- Initial management involves lifestyle interventions focusing on diet, smoking cessation and exercise.
- If this fails to achieve the target, drug therapy is initiated. Treatment options include the biguanide metformin, sulphonyureas such as gliclazide and tobutamide, meglitinides such as repaglinide, thiazolidinediones (glitazones) such as rosiglitazone, and the glucosidase inhibitor acarbose.
- The choice of initial therapy is usually made based on the person's body mass index (BMI).
- The majority of type 2 diabetics are obese, and metformin is recommended in those with a BMI more than 25 unless there is renal impairment or intolerance, where a sulphonylurea may be used.
- If metformin is ineffective a sulphonyurea should be added. If this fails to provide control, the patient should be reviewed by a specialist and the addition of insulin or a glitazone is usually considered.
- In those with a BMI less than 25 a sulphonylurea is usually first-line therapy, with metformin added if targets are not achieved. Again insulin and glitazones are next choices but patients should be referred for review by a specialist.
- Acarbose is usually only used for the treatment of resistant disease or where there is intolerance or contraindications to other drugs.

General management
- Diet management is important in both types of diabetes. Some patients with type 2 may achieve adequate control through appropriate diet without the need for medications. However, all patients will benefit from better dietary control.

Tip

- Meals should be at regular intervals. Carbohydrates should ideally have a low glycaemic index (e.g. wholemeal pasta and bread), rather than be refined.
- Patients should try to limit fat intake, increase fibre and eat at least five portions of fruit and vegetables per day.
- Alcohol and salt intake should be kept within recommended limits: salt 6 g per day for adults and alcohol up to 14 units/week for women and 21 units/week for men.
- Other risk factors for cardiovascular disease should be managed where appropriate, such as hypertension and dyslipidaemias.
- Overall, early and intensive treatment is associated with a decreased risk of the complications of diabetes.

Monitoring parameters

- Overall glycaemic control is measured using HbA1c measurements. Ideally the target should be less than 6.5%, but a more realistic and reasonable target in most patients is 6.5–7.5%. This should be measured every 2–6 months depending on the previous level of control.
- Signs of secondary complications should be assessed through assessment of renal function, blood pressure, urine dipstick testing for presence of protein, foot review, eye tests, weight and waist circumference, fasting blood lipids and liver function tests.
- Changes to drug therapy should be made if glycaemic control is unsatisfactory or the patient is experiencing any drug related problems.
- Each antidiabetic should be monitored for the presence of adverse effects.

Insulin

- Patient's injections should be assessed regularly to ensure they are using insulin appropriately.
- Injection sites should be rotated to avoid reactions, such as lipohypertrophy.
- If the patient is suffering from frequent hyper- or hypoglycaemic episodes, their regimen should be review and adjusted as necessary. It is usual for patient's insulin requirements to increase with time.

Metformin

- Many patients suffer GI complaints with metformin, such as anorexia and diarrhoea. These may be minimised by gradually increasing the dose and taking it with food.

- In some patients, the GI disturbances may be so severe as to prevent patients from continuing the drug.
- There is a risk of lactic acidosis, especially in those with renal or hepatic dysfunction; therefore, regular monitoring of renal and liver function is important.
- Metformin many contribute to renal failure and development of lactic acidosis when used with radiographic contrast dyes so should be omitted for at least 2 days when these are used.

Sulphonylureas

- Unlike metformin, the sulphonylureas may cause hypoglycaemia; therefore, the shorter-acting agents such as gliclazide are preferred.
- Sulphonylureas may induce weight gain, so regular monitoring of weight is important.

Glitazones

- Glitazones may cause oedema, especially in those with cardiac failure. Signs of oedema such as swollen ankles and breathlessness should be looked for.
- Glitazones may cause drug-induced hepatotoxicity, so liver function should be assessed at regular intervals.
- Full blood counts should also be performed as glitazones may induce anaemia.

Counselling

- Patients must be aware of the short- and long-term complications of their disease and the steps they can take to minimise these.
- They must be aware of how each drug should be used and any potential adverse effects.
- Those using insulin will require extensive counselling on the proper use of their insulin device, when to take the dose, the need to rotate injection sites and the storage requirements of their device. Insulin must be stored in the fridge to maintain long-term patency; however, once in use it can be kept out of the fridge for 4–6 weeks depending on the preparation. Insulin should be at room temperature prior to administration.
- Patients should be aware of the signs of hypoglycaemia:
- palpitations and tachycardia
- pallor
- tremor

Tips

Patients receiving treatment for diabetes are entitled to free prescriptions. Many patients are not aware of this or that it applies to all of their prescriptions not only the ones for their antidiabetic medication.

Many patients are worried about the sugar content of liquid medications. It should be explained that the amounts of sugar contained in the major of preparations will do little to alter their overall glycaemic control.

- sweating
- hunger
- headache
- behavioural disturbances, e.g. aggression
- faintness and drowsiness
- loss of concentration
- visual disturbances
- confusion
- coma.

■ Patients and their carers should be aware of the action required if these signs occur. In mild cases, the ingestion of simple sugars (e.g. glucose tablets or drinks) should induce normoglycaemia. Patients should recheck their blood sugars at 15 min intervals to ensure correction. In severe hypoglaecaemia they should seek urgent medical attention.

■ Patients should be aware that during stressful situations, such as surgery and infections, they may require increased monitoring and adjustments to their usual amounts of insulin.

■ All patients should be fully aware of the importance of diet for their glycaemic control.

■ Patients should be aware of how to monitor their diabetes and how often to perform such monitoring. Type 1 diabetics require more intensive monitoring, and the majority will monitor their capillary blood glucose levels at home. They should also have urine test strips to test for ketones when necessary.

■ Those with type 2 diabetes may perform self-testing if they have poor overall control.

■ Patients receiving insulin should be aware of the need to dispose of needles and lancets safely and have appropriate equipment provided.

Multiple choice questions

1. Which of the following is *not* an indication of hypoglycaemia?
a. Sweating
b. Faintness
c. Confusion
d. Bradycardia
e. Drowsiness

2. Are the following statements true or false?
a. Metformin is the first therapy for all type 2 diabetics.
b. Type 1 diabetes is associated with an increased incidence of hypertension and dyslipidaemias.
c. Long-acting insulins may be administered once daily.

d. An HbA1c of 7% would indicate good long-term glycaemic control.
e. Retinopathy and nephropathy are microvascular complications of diabetes.

Useful websites

www.diabetes.org.uk
www.nice.org.uk

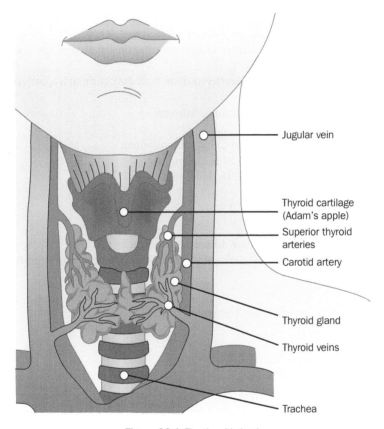

Jugular vein

Thyroid cartilage
(Adam's apple)

Superior thyroid
arteries

Carotid artery

Thyroid gland

Thyroid veins

Trachea

Figure 26.1 The thyroid gland.

Overview

- Hypothyroidism is the deficiency of thyroid hormones.
- There are two types of hypothyroidism: primary and secondary.
- Signs and symptoms of hypothyroidism include bradycardia, lethargy, weight gain and depression.

Tip

Aetiology

- Hypothyroidism is the deficiency of thyroid hormones.
- Primary hypothyroidism is the failure of the thyroid gland.
- Secondary hypothyroidism is when the pituitary fails to secrete thyroid-stimulating hormone (TSH).
- Hashimoto's disease is autoimmune destruction of the thyroid gland.
- Treatment of hyperthyroidism that may induce hypothyroidism includes:
- drugs, e.g. amiodarone, lithium
- radioiodine
- surgical treatment of hyperthyroidism
- iodine replacement in deficiency
- TSH replacement in deficiency.

Epidemiology

- Primary hypothyroidism is common in the UK.
- Women are 20 times more likely to develop hypothyroidism than men.

Signs and symptoms

- Weight gain
- Constipation
- Depression
- Cold intolerance
- Lethargy
- Coarse skin and hair
- Bradycardia
- Brittle nails
- Puffy eyes
- Reduced cognitive function
- Anaemia
- Subfertility.

Investigations

- Simple laboratory investigation of free serum thyroid hormones (triiodothyronine (T_3) and thyroxine (T_4)) and TSH.
- In primary hypothyroidism, TSH levels are noticeably high and free T_3 and T_4 are low.

Management

- Aim of treatment is to replace the hormone to maintain the patient's quality of life.
- Treatment choice is T_4 replacement, e.g. levothyroxine.
- Dose is titrated accordingly to prevent either over- or undertreatment.
- Low doses are given to initiate treatment.
- Higher doses are associated with the development of angina or a myocardial infarction.
- Treatment is lifelong.

Tip

Before replacement therapy is started, check for glucocorticoid deficiency; treatment with thyroxine may induce hypoadrenal crisis if deficiency is present. Corticosteroid therapy should be initiated for glucocorticoid deficiency before starting replacement thyroxine therapy.

Monitoring parameters

- Side-effects of levothyroxine/liothyronine include arrhythmias, diarrhoea, anginal pain, tachycardia, headache and muscle cramp. These side-effects occur with toxic doses.
- Monitoring TSH levels will give a clear indication of the effectiveness of therapy.
- Thyroxine therapy must be used cautiously in patients with cardiovascular disease; baseline ECG should be taken before initiating treatment.
- Patients suffering with diabetes mellitus may need the dosage of their antidiabetic therapy increased.

Tip

Myxoedema coma is life threatening and occurs when hypothyroidism remains untreated.

Counselling

- Treatment is lifelong and should be taken daily.
- Prompt medical advice should be sought if any of the side-effects mentioned are experienced; cardiac side-effects in particular.

Multiple choice questions

1. Which of the following is *not* a side-effect of replacement thyroxine therapy?
a. Palpitation
b. Bradycardia
c. Anginal pain
d. Diarrhoea
e. Arrhythmias

Useful websites

http://www.nhsdirect.nhs.uk
http://clinicalevidence.bmj.com/ceweb/conditions

chapter 27
Hyperthyroidism

Overview

- Hyperthyroidism is the excessive production of thyroid hormones (thyrotoxicosis).
- There are three main treatments available for thyrotoxicosis: drugs, radioiodine and surgery.
- Signs and symptoms include goitre, weight loss and eyelid retraction.

Aetiology

- Hyperthyroidism is the excessive production of thyroid hormones (thyrotoxicosis)
- Causes include
- Grave's disease: the most common cause
- iodine administration
- drugs containing iodine, e.g. amiodarone
- thyroiditis
- excessive triiodothyronine (T_3) and thyroxine (T_4) ingestion
- toxic multinodular goitre.

Epidemiology

Hyperthyroidism is a common condition (approximate prevalence is 2 per 1000), again affecting more women than men.

Signs and symptoms

- Weight loss
- Fatigue
- Sweating
- Insomnia
- Palpitation
- Goitre
- Eyelid retraction
- Muscle weakness
- Angina and heart failure
- Diarrhoea.

Investigations

- Simple biochemical laboratory investigation of free serum thyroid hormones (T_3 and T_4) and thyroid-stimulating hormone (TSH).

- Patients with hyperthyroidism display excessively high levels of T_3 and T_4, and TSH levels are suppressed to subnormal levels.

Management

- Aim of treatment is to restore normal thyroid hormone levels in the body and maintain general patient well-being.
- There are three main treatments available for thyrotoxicosis:
- drug treatment with thionamide, e.g. carbimazole, propylthiouracil
- radioiodine: commonly used in the elderly; most patients will need to be prescribed replacement thyroxine lifelong as hypothyroidism can occur
- surgery: used in patients with very large goitres or for whom drug therapy is contraindicated and radioiodine is not an option.

Tips

Propranolol can be prescribed for rapid relief of thyrotoxic symptoms and can be given concurrently with antithyroid therapy.

There is 10% cross-sensitivity between propylthiouracil and carbimzaole; patients can be changed between these if adverse effects occur with one.

Monitoring parameters

- Side-effects of carbimazole and propylthiouracil include nausea, GI disturbances, alopecia, agranulocytosis and neutropenia, jaundice and bone marrow suppression.
- In addition to the above, other side-effects of propylthiouracil include thrombocytopenia, nephritis and hepatitis.
- Clinicians should be able to recognise potential bone marrow suppression (rash, signs of infection anywhere in the body, sore throat) and a full blood count should be carried out.
- Carbimazole/propylthiouracil should be stopped immediately if bone marrow suppression/neutropenia is suspected.
- Thyroid function tests should be carried out to monitor treatment (all three types of treatment).

Counselling

- Patients should watch out for signs of infection such as sore throat, high temperature or malaise, and seek immediate medical advice.
- Side-effects of the drugs prescribed should be explained.
- Patients must understand the need for regular reviews.

Multiple choice questions

1. Which of the following is *not* a symptom or sign of hyperthyroidism?
a. Weight loss
b. Goitre

c. Fatigue
d. Coarse hair
e. Angina

Useful websites

http://www.nhsdirect.nhs.uk
http://clinicalevidence.bmj.com/ceweb/conditions

The skin

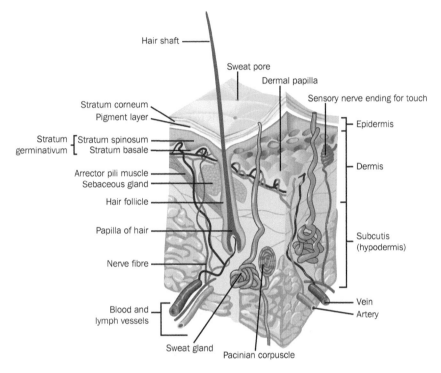

Hair shaft

Sweat pore

Dermal papilla

Sensory nerve ending for touch

Stratum corneum
Pigment layer

Epidermis

Stratum germinativum [Stratum spinosum
Stratum basale

Dermis

Arrector pili muscle
Sebaceous gland

Hair follicle

Papilla of hair

Subcutis (hypodermis)

Nerve fibre

Blood and lymph vessels

Vein
Artery

Sweat gland

Pacinian corpuscle

Figure 28.1 The skin.

Overview

- Eczema is an inflammatory skin disorder.
- Topical corticosteroids and emollients are used for its treatment.

What is eczema?

- Eczema is an inflammatory skin disorder.
- The main types are atopic eczema and contact dermatitis.
- Other types include seborrhoeic, discoid, varicose and asteatotic eczema.

Tip

The term dermatitis can also be used instead of eczema.

■ Swelling of the epidermis by oedema causes formation of tiny vesicles, which can enlarge and rupture leading to inflammation of both the dermis and the epidermis.

Atopic eczema

■ Atopic eczema can be linked to family history, environment or immunological factors.
■ Sufferers have prolonged hypersensitivity to pollen, dust mite (common antigens in the environment).
■ 25–50% of sufferers will develop asthma or hayfever.
■ Symptoms in infancy are acute and involve the face and trunk.
■ In childhood, the rash tends to be on the back of the knees, fronts of elbows, wrists and ankles.
■ In adulthood, lichenification is a characteristic. Rash would develop on the face and trunk.
■ Factors causing atopic eczema include:
— dryness
— hot temperatures
— irritants: soap and water
— stress
— infection.

Contact dermatitis

■ Contact dermatitis is a delayed hypersensitivity reaction to allergens.
■ Patch testing is used to confirm an allergy.

■ Common allergens causing contact dermatitis include:
— rubber compounds (such as domestic rubber gloves)
— plants
— resins
— plastic
— cosmetics
— nickel (present in jewellery)

Tip

The patient should avoid the allergen once cause is established. Hypersensitivity to the allergen is lifelong and can aggravate dermatitis if patient has further contact.

— cement
— leather
— hair dye
— perfume
— topical medication (such as neomycin, lidocaine).

Signs and symptoms

Acute signs include:

- pruritis
- red, hot and swelling
- crusting
- exudation
- scaling.

Chronic signs include those for acute eczema plus:

- painful fissures
- scratch marks
- lichenification.

Investigations

- Patch tests are carried out in suspected cases of contact dermatitis.
- Prick tests are carried out to diagnose atopic eczema.
- IgE is occasionally measured to diagnose atopic eczema and the causative allergen.

Management

- Treatment is similar for all types of eczema:
- *emollients* (e.g. aqueous cream): hydrate the skin and can be used as a heavy moisturiser or soap
- *topical corticosteroids* (e.g. hydrocortisone 1% cream) is used as an anti-inflammatory agent
- *systemic corticosteroids* (e.g. prednisolone) can be used short term to reduce inflammation in acute exacerbations
- *potassium permanganate crystals* added to the bath can be used for weeping eczema
- *Tacrolimus* and *pimecrolimus* are topical immunosuppressants recently used for the treatment of eczema.
- In severe eczema, *ciclosporin* (a narrow therapeutic drug) can be used; patients need to be monitored for signs of infection and they should avoid drinking grapefruit juice while taking ciclosporin.

Monitoring parameters

- Using emollients appropriately will decrease the requirement for topical steroids; patients should be using emollients regularly
- Adequate quantities of emollients should be supplied.
- Side-effects of topical corticosteroids include thinning of the skin, striae and susceptibility to skin infections. Some systemic absorption can lead to pituitary adrenal axis suppression and cushingnoid features.

Tip

Counselling

- Emollient creams, not soap, should be used to wash the face and to shower, and emollient oils are used in the bath.
- Steroid creams should be applied thinly, as they may cause thinning of the skin. They should not be used as an emollient.
- There are four different potencies of steroids. Usually the highest tolerable potency is given to control a flare up of eczema and a lower potency is given to maintain control.
- Antihistamines may be prescribed if itching is causing distress to the patient.

Multiple choice questions

1. Which of the following is *not* a common allergen causing contact dermatitis?
a. Hydrocortisone
b. Nickel
c. Neomycin
d. Leather
e. Rubber gloves

2. Are the following statements true or false?
a. Patch tests are used in contact dermatitis.
b. Stress can contribute to atopic eczema.
c. Pruritis is a chronic symptom.
d. Eczema is an inflammatory disorder.

Useful website

http://www.nhsdirect.nhs.uk

chapter 29

Psoriasis

Overview

- Psoriasis is a chronic condition affecting the skin and joints.
- Red, scaly plaques occur on the skin.
- Many factors can aggravate the condition, such as drugs, stress or infections.
- Treatment aims are to keep the condition at bay.
- Many topical and systemic preparations are available to help to reduce the symptoms and control the condition.

What is psoriasis?

- Psoriasis affects the skin and joints.
- The condition is caused by rapid proliferation of epidermal cells; cell turnover is increased to 2–6 days compared with the usual turnover of 28–30 days.
- Inflammatory arthritis may develop.
- Causes include:
- family history
- infection; upper respiratory tract in particular
- drugs, e.g. lithium, beta-blockers
- stress
- skin injury, e.g. cut, burn, scar
- alcohol
- smoking.
- There are many different types of psoriasis. These include:
- chronic plaque psoriasis: medium to large plaques
- guttate psoriasis: multiple small plaques all over the body
- psoriasis of the nails, scalp, palms and soles
- flexural psoriasis: occurs in the groin, genitalia
- erythrodermic pustular psoriasis: uncommon and may be life threatening; it occurs all over body and there is general malaise
- arthritic psoriasis: affecting the joints.

Signs and symptoms

- Red scaly lesions
- Silver scales on the skin
- Plaque formation
- Affects mainly knees, hands, elbows, scalp.

Management

- *Emollients* (e.g. aqueous cream) hydrate the skin and are used as a heavy moisturiser or soap.
- *Topical corticosteroids* (e.g. hydrocortisone 1% cream) are used as anti-inflammatory agents.
- *Dithranol* decreases cell division and heals plaques. Dithranol can stain the skin and clothing and may be inappropriate for use in the home for this reason.
- *Coal tar* is cytostatic; it enhances healing if used in conjunction with ultraviolet B in phototherapy treatment.
- *Phototherapy* can be used with ultraviolet B or as PUVA (psoralen plus ultraviolet A) for severe psoriasis.
- *Vitamin D analogues* (e.g. calcipotriol) are more effective than coal tar. Calcipotriol should not be used on the face as it may cause irritation. Excessive use can precipitate hypercalcaemia.
- *Methotrexate* is used for arthritic psoriasis and severe psoriasis.
- *Retinoids* (e.g. vitamin A; retinol) are used for severe resistant psoriasis.
- *Ciclosporin* is used for severe psoriasis.
- *Cytokine inhibitors* (e.g. infliximab) are used in moderate to severe psoriasis.

Tips

Lotions and topical applications may be ineffective on the scalp. A keratolytic (salicyclic acid) should be applied first.

Potent steroids are recommended for the hands and feet.

Monitoring

- Lesions are monitored to see if the preparations are improving or worsening the condition.
- Ciclosporin: has a narrow therapeutic index and so the drug requires monitoring: renal function and blood pressure. Grapefruit juice must be avoided as this can interfere with the metabolism of ciclosporin.
- Retinoids may cause abnormalities in liver function tests and plasma lipids; dry skin and alopecia are frequently seen side-effects.
- Methotrexate is given as a once weekly dose; toxicity can occur if it is used with other drugs that reduce its excretion (e.g. NSAIDs). Side-effects include nausea, blood disorders, liver toxicity, GI bleeding. These should be monitored closely.

Counselling

- Emollient creams, not soap, are used to wash the face and to shower and emollient oils are used in the bath.
- Steroid creams should be applied thinly as they may cause thinning of the skin. They should not be used as an emollient.
- Factors that aggravate the condition should be avoided.

Multiple choice questions

1. Which of the following is *not* usually used for the management of psoriasis?
a. Methotrexate
b. Coal tar
c. Ciclosporin
d. PUVA
e. Propranolol

2. Are the following statements regarding psoriasis true or false?
a. Psoriasis may affect the joints.
b. Symptoms include plaque formation.
c. Psoriasis may affect the nails.
d. Grapefruit juice can be consumed with ciclosporin therapy.

Useful website

http://www.nhsdirect.nhs.uk

The eye

chapter 30
Glaucoma

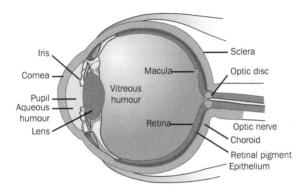

Figure 30.1 The eye.

Overview

- Glaucoma is characterised by raised intraocular pressure.
- It is usually asymptomatic.
- Age, race, family history and diabetes are risk factors.
- Aim of treatment is to reduce intraocular pressure.

Aetiology

- Glaucoma is a range of disorders usually characterised by raised intraocular pressure and leading to damage of the optic nerve.
- Damage to the optic nerve can occur with a normal intraocular pressure.
- Glaucoma can be classified as primary or secondary.
- Primary glaucoma includes primary open-angle glaucoma (chronic simple glaucoma), the most common form of glaucoma, and primary angle-closure glaucoma.
- Primary open-angle glaucoma is caused by blockage in the trabecular meshwork, which drains the anterior chamber of the eye to the episcleral veins through the canal Schlemm.
- Primary angle-closure glaucoma is generally acute in onset and may require treatment as a medical emergency.
- Primary angle-closure glaucoma results from decreased outflow of aqueous humour, causing accumulation of fluid in the eye.

- Secondary glaucomas can result from a wide range of causes, such as inflammation, tumours or congenital abnormalities.

As primary open-angle glaucoma is the most common form of glaucoma, this chapter will primarily focus on this type.

Tip

In the UK, those aged over 40 years with an immediate family member diagnosed with glaucoma are entitled to free annual sight tests.

Epidemiology

Risk factors associated with primary open-angle glaucoma are:

- age: glaucoma affects 2 in 100 over the age of 40 and 1 in 10 over the age of 70 years
- race: those of African origin have greater incidence, earlier onset and greater severity
- family: 10% likelihood of first-degree relatives developing glaucoma
- short sight: those affected are prone to glaucoma
- diabetes: believed to increase the risk of developing glaucoma.

Signs and symptoms

- Glaucoma is usually asymptomatic, unless it is in the advanced stages.
- Symptoms include worsening of vision.
- Signs include raised intraocular pressure and increased variation in intraocular pressure.

Investigations

- Most patients are diagnosed at routine eye appointments:
- intraocular pressure measured by tonometry
- appearance of the optic nerve by ophthalmoscopy
- peripheral vision assessment using perimetry (spot testing).
- It is important that all three tests are carried out to confirm diagnosis.

Management

- Aim of treatment is to reduce intraocular pressure.
- Five main classes of drug are used for treatment of glaucoma; all work by reducing intraocular pressure by different mechanisms:
- *beta-blockers* (e.g. timolol, levobunolol) reduce aqueous humour production
- *prostaglandin analogues* (e.g. latanoprost) increase uveoscleral outflow

- *sympathomimetics* (e.g. brimodine) improve drainage through the trabecular meshwork and decrease aqueous production by stimulation of α_2-adrenoceptors
- *carbonic anhydrase inhibitors* (e.g. dorzolamide) reduce aqueous humour production
- *miotics* (e.g. pilocarpine) are usually given for acute glaucoma to increase drainage through the trabecular meshwork.
- Topical beta-blockers or prostaglandin analogues are first choice.

Monitoring parameters

- Tonometry, ophthalmoscopy and perimetry should be monitored for effectiveness of treatment.
- Systemic absorption of beta-blockers may occur; therefore, they are contraindicated in asthma, chronic obstructive pulmonary disease, and uncontrolled heart failure, bradycardia and heart block. Systemic side-effects are described in the cardiovascular section.

> **Tip**
> Although rare, systemic side-effects may occur in susceptible individuals with any of the five classes of drug.

- Local adverse effects of beta-blockers include ocular stinging, burning, itching, pain, erythema, dry eyes and allergic reactions.
- Changes in eye coloration should be monitored with prostaglandin analogue therapy as brown pigmentation may occur
- Local side-effects of prostaglandin analogues include thickening and lengthening of eye lashes, blepharitis, ocular irritation and pain, and congunctival hyperaemia.
- Sympathomimetics have local side-effects including conjunctival hyperaemia, burning, stinging, pruritis and visual disturbances.
- Carbonic anhydrase inhibitors can cause local burning, itching, blurred vision, tearing, conjunctivitis, ocular discharge and eye lid pain.
- Miotics can cause blurred vision, allergic conjunctivitis, lens changes, myopia, pain and ciliary spasm. Headache commonly occurs, especially in the first 2–4 weeks of treatment.

Counselling

> **Tip**
> If more than one preparation is being used, they should be administered at least 10 min apart.

- Patients should wash their hands before putting in eye drops.
- They should not allow the tip of the container to touch their eyes or areas around the eye.

- Contamination with bacteria can cause eye infections, potentially causing loss of vision.
- When advising on the administration of eye drops, the following points should be covered:
- tilt head back and pull the lower eyelid down slightly to form a pocket between the eyelid and eye
- invert the container and press lightly with thumb and forefinger until a single drop is instilled into the eye
- replace the cap immediately after use.

Multiple choice questions

1. Which of the following is *not* a risk factor for primary open-angle glaucoma?
a. Age
b. Sex
c. Race
d. Family history
e. Diabetes

2. Are the following statements true or false?
a. Beta-blockers reduce intraocular pressure by reducing aqueous humour production.
b. Beta-blocker eye drops are safe for use in patients with hypertension.
c. Beta-blockers may cause systemic side-effects in patients using local eye drops.
d. Beta-blocker eye drops are used as second-line treatment in glaucoma.

Useful websites

http://www.rnib.org.uk
http://www.nhsdirect.nhs.uk

Musculoskeletal disorders

chapter 31

Rheumatoid arthritis

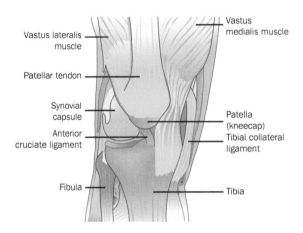

Vastus lateralis muscle

Vastus medialis muscle

Patellar tendon

Synovial capsule

Patella (kneecap)

Anterior cruciate ligament

Tibial collateral ligament

Fibula

Tibia

Overview

- Rheumatoid arthritis is a chronic systemic autoimmune disorder that most commonly causes inflammation and tissue damage in joints and tendon sheaths.
- Diagnostic criteria are based on the American Rheumatism Association criteria.
- Various pain relief and anti-inflammatory drugs can be given to reduce the pain and inflammation (e.g. NSAIDs, paracetamol).
- Disease modifying antirheumatic drugs (DMARDs) slow down disease progression and maintain remission.
- Counselling patients with rheumatoid arthritis is paramount, including educating about the disease and the drugs used.

Aetiology

- Rheumatoid arthritis is a chronic inflammatory condition affecting joints.
- No single factor has been highlighted as the cause for the disease.
- Risk factors include:
- smoking
- family history
- female sex.

Epidemiology

- 1% of the population worldwide is affected by rheumatoid arthritis.
- Females are at higher risk of having the condition.
- The average age of developing the condition is 65 years.

Signs and symptoms

Rheumatoid arthritis is a systemic disease with both articular and non-articular symptoms:

- anorexia
- weight loss
- fatigue
- osteoporosis
- symmetrical swelling of joints
- swan neck deformity of the fingers
- deformity of thumb
- morning stiffness.

Diagnostic criteria

Criteria for the diagnosis of rheumatoid arthritis have been developed by the American Rheumatism Association (Table 31.1).[1] If the patient presents with four or more of the criteria, a diagnosis of rheumatoid arthritis can be confirmed.

Investigations

- Diagnosis is confirmed using the American Rheumatism Association criteria plus biochemical investigations for markers that confirm an inflammatory condition:
- — ESR
- — CRP
- — rheumatoid factor (RF)

Tip

Absence of a high rheumatoid factor titre does not rule out rheumatoid arthritis as the factor is only present in 60–70% of patients.

Table 31.1 American Rheumatism Association criteria for the diagnosis of rheumatoid arthritis

Criteria	Comment
Morning stiffness	Lasting for more than an hour for more than 6 weeks
Arthritis of three or more joint areas	Soft tissue swelling or exudation for more than 6 weeks
Arthritis of hand joints	Swelling for more than 6 weeks
Symmetrical arthritis	Symmetry of same joint areas on both sides of the body for more than 6 weeks
Rheumatoid nodules	
Serum rheumatoid factor	
Radiographic changes	

- anti-nuclear antibodies (ANA)
- plasma viscosity (PV).
- Radiography of hands and feet will demonstrate signs of erosion.

Management

Aim of treatment is to relieve symptoms, suppress inflammation, preserve and improve functional ability and maintain a normal lifestyle.

- *Physiotherapy* strengthens joints and helps to reduce pain.
- *Electrotherapy* helps to reduce swelling and controls symptoms.
- *Occupational therapy* educates patients on how to protect their joints and live with the condition.
- Simple *analgesia* (e.g. paracetamol) is used as an adjunct to manage pain.
- The *NSAIDs* (e.g. ibuprofen, naproxen) reduce pain and stiffness by inhibiting prostaglandins produced by cyclo-oxygenases I and II. Cyclo-oxygenase II is responsible for mediating pain and inflammation.
- *Disease modifying antirheumatic drugs* (DMARDs, e.g. methotrexate, sulfasalazine) suppress disease and induce and maintain remission. Prescribing DMARDS early is recommended. Two or more DMARDs can be prescribed together to produce a desired effect, e.g. methotrexate plus sufasalazine or ciclosporin plus hydroxychloroquine. Response rates for DMARDs are approximately 60%. Cytokine inhibitors can be used in non-responsive patients.
- *Corticosteroids* suppress cytokines and can elicit signs of rapid improvement in the disease. They are potent anti-inflammatory agents and can be given orally long term or as cover until a DMARD takes effect, or intra-articularly every few weeks. Intra-articular injections can be used for rapid symptomatic relief but should not be given more than three times in a year to any one joint.
- *Cytokine inhibitors* (anti-tumour necrosis factor (TNF), e.g. infliximab, etanercept) have their main site of action in the inflammatory pathway, which is modulated by cytokines such as TNF. Anti-TNFs are prescribed concomitantly with methotrexate and are given by slow IV infusion. Cytokine inhibitors should be used under specialist supervision; for individual profiles see BNF Section 10.1.3. Guidelines for the use of anti-TNFs in rheumatoid arthritis were published by NICE in 2002.

Tips

Simple analgesics should be used instead of NSAIDs if pain is well controlled with a simple analgesic.

If patients are taking NSAIDs or DMARDs over a long period, a gastroprotective agent such as a proton pump inhibitor may need to be prescribed.

Monitoring parameters

- Pain score questionnaires will assess the extent of pain patients are feeling when carrying out certain tasks.
- Radiography monitors disease progression and remission.
- A full blood count should include all inflammatory markers (e.g. CRP, ESR, RF).
- The lowest possible dose of NSAID should be prescribed to minimise toxicity.
- NSAID side-effects include:
- dyspepsia
- gastric erosions
- peptic ulceration
- small bowel inflammation and bleeding
- haematemesis or melaena
- GI blood loss
- anaemia.
- Renal function should be monitored as renal toxicity can occur.
- Side-effects of corticosteroids include:
- osteoporosis
- hypertension
- glaucoma
- diabetes
- weight gain
- Cushing effect
- adrenal suppression
- depression.
- Cytokine inhibitors should be used under specialist supervision.
- Side-effects of cytokine inhibitors include:
- chest pain
- drowsiness
- constipation
- cough
- sore throat
- tremor
- dizziness.
- Patients should be evaluated for tuberculosis.
- Table 31.2 gives the adverse effects and monitoring parameters for DMARDs.[2]

Counselling

- The patient needs to be educated about the disease.
- External help (e.g. from occupational therapists) should be discussed and a referral made if necessary.

Table 31.2 Profiles of disease modifying antirheumatic drugs (DMARDs)

DMARD	Common/minor adverse effects	Rare/severe adverse effects	Monitoring parameters	Advantages
Hydroxychloroquine	Nausea, headaches	Retinal toxicity	Eye check Reduce dose if renal impairment	No blood monitoring required. Can use when uncertain of diagnosis (e.g. inflammatory arthritis, connective tissue disease). Can use despite leucopenia or thrombocytopenia
Sulfasalazine	Nausea, diarrhoea, headache, mouth ulcers, rash, oligospermia (reversible), staining of soft contact lenses, abnormal LFTs	Leucopenia	FBC, LFT, renal function, urinalysis	Rapid onset action (8–12 weeks). Can use when uncertain of diagnosis (e.g. reactive/psoriatic/RA). Relatively safe in thrombocytopenia
Methotrexate	Nausea, diarrhoea, mouth ulcers, rash, alopecia, abnormal LFTs	Leucopenia/ thrombocytopenia, pneumonitis, sepsis, liver disease (late), nodulosis, Epstein–Barr virus associated-lymphoma	FBC, LFT, renal function Advise to restrict alcohol intake	Rapid onset action (6–10 weeks). Can use when uncertain of diagnosis (e.g. RA, psoriatic/connective tissue disease). Can be given orally, IM or SC. Weekly administration
IM gold	Mouth ulcers, rash, nitritoid reactions	Thrombocytopenia/ leucopenia, proteinuria, colitis	FBC, LFT, renal function, urinalysis	Patient preference ensures compliance

Table 31.2 (continued)

Penicillamine	Nausea/loss of taste, dose-related, reversible fall in platelet count	Proteinuria, late autoimmune disease	FBC, U&E, urinalysis	
Auranofin	Diarrhoea	Leucopenia	FBC, renal function, urinalysis	Oral gold option
Azathioprine	Nausea	Leucopenia, sepsis, lymphoma (late)	FBC, LFT	Can be used in patients with renal disease
Leflunomide,	Alopecia, diarrhoea, nausea, rash	Leucopenia, hepatitis, thrombocytopenia	FBC, LFT, renal function, BP monitoring	Remain to be established (recently introduced)
Ciclosporin	Paraesthesia/tremor/ headaches, hypertrichosis, gingival hypertrophy, nausea	Hypertension, renal disease, sepsis	LFT, renal function, BP monitoring	

RA, rheumatoid arthritis; FBC, full blood count; LFT, liver function tests; BP, blood pressure, U&E, urea and electrolytes.
Adapted from Scottish Intercollegiate Guidelines Network (2001)[2]

- NSAIDs to be taken with or after food to protect the stomach.
- Side-effects of drugs prescribed should be explained.
- A named healthcare professional should be linked to chronic sufferers for reporting of side-effects or worsening symptoms.
- It is important that patients keep their appointments at the hospital/rheumatology clinic; drugs are monitored for toxicity and efficacy and the importance of adhering to the appointments should be discussed.
- Patients should be reminded not to buy NSAIDs or paracetamol over the counter if they are taking long-term NSAIDs or paracetamol for rheumatoid arthritis.

Multiple choice questions

1. Which of the following is *not* a side-effect of NSAIDs?
a. Gastric bleeding
b. Anaemia
c. Dyspepsia
d. Dyspnoea
e. Renal toxicity

2. Are the following statements true or false?
a. Rheumatoid arthritis is an acute disease.
b. Night-time waking is a common sign of rheumatoid arthritis.
c. Men are more at risk of developing the disease than women.
d. Infliximab is an anti-TNF and inhibits cytokines in the inflammatory pathway.

References

1. Arnett FC *et al.* (1988). The American Rheumatism Association 1987 revised criteria for the classification of rheumatoid arthritis. *Arthritis Rheum* 31:315–324.
2. Scottish Intercollegiate Guidelines Network (2001). *Management of Early Rheumatoid Arthritis*. [SIGN Publication No. 48.] Edinburgh: Scottish Intercollegiate Guidelines Network.

Useful websites

http://www.rheumatoid.org.uk/
http://www.nhsdirect.nhs.uk
http://www.sign.ac.uk/guidelines
http://www.nice.org.uk

chapter 32

Osteoarthritis

Overview

- Osteoarthritis is a disease of the synovial joints.
- There are a variety of risk factors associated with the condition, including obesity and family history.
- Symptoms include stiffness, loss of fuction and muscle wasting.
- Radiography and MRI can help to confirm the diagnosis.
- Patients are advised to exercise and to reduce weight in order to decrease the burden on the body.
- Treatment includes simple paracetamol with topical or systemic NSAIDs.

Aetiology

- Osteoarthritis is a disease of the synovial joints.
- *Risk factors* include:
- family history
- obesity
- age
- trauma
- joint shape
- physical and occupation factors.
- A variety of insults can contribute to damage of the synovial joints.

Epidemiology

- Osteoarthritis is the most common form of arthritis.
- 2% of individuals less than 45 years of age suffer with osteoarthritis; in people over 65 years, 68% women and 58% men are affected.

Signs and symptoms

- Joint pain
- Stiffness
- Loss of function
- Joint tenderness
- Muscle wasting
- Swelling of joints
- Commonly affected joints are knees, hips, cervical, lumbar spine, distal interphalangeal joints.

Tip

Investigations

- Diagnosis is made on the clinical presentation.
- Radiography shows abnormalities in advanced stages only.
- MRI can highlight early cartilage changes.
- Blood tests are normal for inflammatory markers: ESR and CRP.
- Rheumatoid factor is negative.

Tips

Management

- Aim of treatment is to reduce pain, increase mobility, reduce disability and slow down disease progression.
- Obese patients should be counselled for weight loss and those who require medication to aid weight loss should be referred.
- Regular paracetamol is used for pain.
- Topical and/or oral NSAIDs can be added.
- Topical capsaicin can be of use for the knee and hand.
- Intra-articular steroid injections can be used for moderate to severe pain.
- If paracetamol and NSAIDs are ineffective in relieving the pain, opioids may be prescribed.
- Joint surgery is an option if the patient has been offered all the pharmacological and non-pharmacological treatments mentioned *and* has joint symptoms that are significantly affecting quality of life.

Monitoring parameters

- Pain score questionaires can assess the level and location of pain, and therapy can then be adjusted at need (Table 32.1).

Table 32.1 Examples of adjusting analgesia based on the severity of pain

Example	Adjustment
1. A patient taking regular paracetamol is complaining of pain in the knees	Add a topical NSAID
2. A patient taking regular paracetamol, regular NSAID and an opioid has been pain free for 6 months	Gradually reduce and stop the opioid and re-evaluate pain

- If NSAIDS are being used, the patient should be monitored for signs of bleeding/ulceration. With regular NSAID treatment, a proton pump inhibitor can be considered.
- Paracetamol should be at a maximum dosage of 4 g in 24 h.

Counselling

- Patients should be counselled on lifestyle changes especially weight loss and the importance of exercise.
- Patients should be aware of the side-effects of the drugs they are taking and report any disturbing side-effects to their pharmacist or doctor.
- Accurate verbal and written information is recommended to improve understanding of osteoarthritis and its management.
- Advice should be offered on appropriate footwear for people with lower limb osteoarthritis.

Tips

Patients should be screened for depression as the condition affects the patient's quality of life.

A holistic approach should be taken when treating osteoarthritis. The patient's function, quality of life, mood, occupation, relationships and extracurricular activities should be discussed and considered.

Multiple choice questions

1. **Which of the following is *not* a sign or symptom of osteoarthritis?**
a. Joint pain
b. Stiffness on waking
c. Tiredness
d. Swelling of joints
e. Wasting of muscles

2. **Are the following statements true or false?**
a. Surgery should be offered to all patients with osteoarthritis.
b. Patients should be encouraged to lose weight.
c. Regular paracetamol is the mainstay of treatment.
d. MRI is useful in diagnosing the condition.

Useful website

http://www.nice.org.uk

Overview

- Gout is a metabolic disorder affecting the joints; the joint of the big toe is usually involved.
- Crystal deposits of uric acid react with the joints to cause inflammation, pain and swelling.
- Acute attacks are treated with NSAIDs or colchicine.
- Chronic treatment comprises hypouricaemic agents or uricosuric agents.

Aetiology

- Gout is a metabolic disorder that is characterised by recurrent acute attacks to the joints.
- Joints react to the deposits of uric acid, an end-product of purine metabolism.
- Overproduction or underexcretion of uric acid can precipitate gout.
- Certain drugs can also be a precipitating factor, such as diuretics.
- Foods high in purine content (e.g. meat, chicken, fish, liver) can aggravate gout.
- Lifestyle can contribute to gout, for example being overweight, overconsumption of alcohol.
- The joint affected is most commonly the joint of the big toe. Other joints, such as wrist and ankle, can also be affected.

> **Tips**
>
> Moderate consumption of wine has not been shown to increase the risk of gout.
> Obesity, excessive alcohol consumption and fasting may lead to hyperuricaemia.

Epidemiology

- Environment: there is a high incidence in New Zealand.
- Sex: there is a strong male preponderance; 95% occurs in men.
- Genetic: an inherited defect in an enzyme of uric acid excretion can occur.
- Age: prevalence increases with age. The peak age group for developing gout is 40–50 years.

Signs and symptoms

- Intense joint pain
- Joint redness
- Extreme tenderness
- Inflammation.

> **Tips**
>
> Symptoms are acute, occurring almost always at night.
> Wearing tight shoes and physical stress (walking uphill) can predispose to acute gout attacks.

Tip

Investigations

Microscopic examination of aspiration from the synovial joint will show monosodium urate crystal deposits.

Management

The aim of treatment is to relieve symptoms, treat the acute attack, prevent further attacks and reduce serum urate levels.

Acute attacks

- NSAIDs are the treatment of choice, especially indometacin; these reduce inflammation and pain.
- Colchicine has an anti-inflammatory effect in the gouty joints; higher doses can give rise to toxicity.
- Steroids can be given intra-articularly or systemically as an alternative to NSAIDs or colchicine.

Tip

Chronic gout

- Allopurinol is a hypouricaemic agent and is first-line therapy in the management of chronic gout.
- Uricosuric agents (e.g. probenecid, sulfinpyrazone) compete with uric acid for reabsorption in the distal convoluted tubule in the kidneys.

Monitoring parameters

- NSAIDs should be administered within 48 h of an acute episode. Side-effects include GI discomfort (occasionally bleeding), angioedema, bronchospasm and headache.
- NSAIDs should be used with caution in patients with a history of hypersensitivity to aspirin or other NSAIDs, in patients with renal impairment (as NSAIDs can cause a decline in renal function).
- NSAIDs are contraindicated in patients with severe heart failure.
- Colchicine can cause nausea, vomiting and abdominal pain; toxic effects include diarrhoea, GI haemorrhage, renal and hepatic damage.
- Allopurinol is well tolerated and has a long half life. Side-effects include rashes, hypersensitivity reactions (e.g. fever, arthralgia) and, rarely, blood disorders and gynaecomastia.

■ The uricosuric agent probenicid is unlicensed for use in the UK but is available on a named-patient basis. Care must be taken for potential interactions with NSAIDs: probenecid increases plasma indometacin, ketoprofen, naproxen and aspirin levels. Side-effects include GI disturbances, urinary frequency, headache, alopecia, haemolytic anemia and sore gums.

Counselling

■ Patients should be advised to decrease beef, pork, lamb and seafood consumption.
■ Foods which have low fat dairy produce (e.g. skimmed milk) are recommended.
■ Alcohol intake should be decreased, especially beer as it adds calories as well as alcohol.
■ Weight should be reduced if obese.
■ Fasting can lead to hyperuricaemia.
■ NSAIDs should be taken at the first sign of an attack. Patients are advised to carry their NSAIDs with them.
■ NSAIDs should be taken with food to minimise GI side-effects.
■ For analgesic or antipyretic purposes, aspirin should be avoided and an alternative, such as paracetamol, used.
■ Allopurinol therapy must be continued regardless and not be stopped despite the patient being asymptomatic.
■ Side-effects of all the drugs and any potential risks should be carefully explained.
■ Adequate fluid intake should be maintained. Current recommendations are 2–3 L per day.

> **Tip**
>
> Aspirin should be avoided in patients suffering with gout as it can worsen an acute attack. Aspirin competes with uric acid for excretion and, therefore, causes an accumulation of uric acid.

Multiple choice questions

1. Which of the following *does not* increase the risk of gout?
a. Wine
b. Pork
c. Aspirin
d. Prawns
e. Bendroflumethiazide

2. Are the following statements true or false?
a. The recommended fluid intake is 1 L per day.
b. Ethambutol can precipitate gout.

c. Allopurinol therapy should be continued regardless of whether symptoms are present or not.
d. Colchicine can be given in an acute situation.

Useful website

http://www.nhsdirect.nhs.uk

Multiple choice answers

Chapter 1

1. **a.** True.
   b. True.
   c. True.
   d. True.
2. **a.** True.
   b. True.
   c. False.
   d. True.

Chapter 2

1. **c**
2. **a.** True.
   b. True.
   c. False.
   d. True.

Chapter 3

1. **c**
2. **a.** True.
   b. True.
   c. False.
   d. True.

Chapter 4

1. **a.** True.
   b. False.
   c. False.
   d. True.
   e. False.

Chapter 5

1. **c**
2. **a.** False.
   b. True.
   c. False.
   d. True.
   e. True.

Chapter 6

1. **d**
2. **a.** False.
   b. False.
   c. False.
   d. True.
   e. False.

Chapter 7

1. **c**
2. **a.** True.
   b. False.
   c. True.
   d. False.

Chapter 8

1. **a, b, e**
2. **a.** True.
   b. True.
   c. True.
   d. True.

Chapter 9

1. **a.** False.
   b. True.
   c. True.
   d. False.
2. **a.** True.
   b. True.
   c. True.

d. False.
e. True.

Chapter 10

1. **c**
2. **a.** True.
   b. True.
   c. False.
   d. False.

Chapter 11

1. **a.** True.
   b. False.
   c. False.
   d. False.
2. **a.** True.
   b. False.
   c. True.
   d. True.
   e. True.

Chapter 12

1. **a**
2. **a.** False.
   b. False.
   c. False.
   d. True.

Chapter 13

1. **c**
2. **a.** True.
   b. False.
   c. True.
   d. True.

Chapter 14

1. d
2. a. False.
   b. True.
   c. True.
   d. False.

Chapter 15

1. a
2. a. True.
   b. True.
   c. True.
   d. True.

Chapter 16

1. a. False.
   b. True.
   c. True.
   d. True.
2. a. False.
   b. False.
   c. True.
   d. False.
   e. False.

Chapter 17

1. c
2. a. False.
   b. True.
   c. True.
   d. False.
   e. True.

Chapter 18

1. b
2. a. False.
   b. True.
   c. True.
   d. True.
   e. False.

Chapter 19

1. b
2. a. False.
   b. False.
   c. True.
   d. True.

Chapter 20

1. b, d, e
2. a. False.
   b. True.
   c. True.
   d. False.
   e. True.

Chapter 21

1. a
2. a. False.
   b. False.
   c. True.
   d. True.
   e. False.

Chapter 22

1. d
2. a. True.
   b. False.
   c. False.
   d. True.
   e. True.

Chapter 23

1. b
2. a. False.
   b. False.
   c. True.
   d. False.
   e. False.

Chapter 24

1. b
2. a. False.
   b. True.
   c. True.
   d. True.

Chapter 25

1. d
2. a. False.
   b. True.
   c. True.
   d. True.
   e. True.

Chapter 26

1. b Bradycardia is a
   symptom of
   hypothyroidism not
   a side-effect of
   replacement
   therapy.

Chapter 27

1. d Coarse hair is a sign/
   symptom of
   hypothryroidism

Chapter 28

1. a
2. a. True.
   b. True.
   c. False.
   d. True.

Chapter 29

1. e
2. a. True.
   b. True.
   c. True.
   d. False.

Chapter 30

1. **b**
2. **a.** True.
   b. True.
   c. True.
   d. False.

Chapter 31

1. **d**

2. **a.** False.
   b. False.
   c. False.
   d. True.

Chapter 32

1. **c**
2. **a.** False.
   b. True.

   c. True.
   d. True.

Chapter 33

1. **a**
2. **a.** False.
   b. True.
   c. True.
   d. True.

Index